Frank G. Holz · Steffen Schmitz-Valckenberg · Richard F. Spaide · Alan C. Bird

Atlas of Fundus Autofluorescence Imaging

Frank G. Holz · Steffen Schmitz-Valckenberg
Richard F. Spaide · Alan C. Bird (Eds.)

Atlas of Fundus Autofluorescence Imaging

With 132 Figures and 1 Table

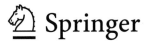

Prof. Dr. med. Frank G. Holz
Department of Ophthalmology
University of Bonn
Ernst-Abbe-Str. 2
53127 Bonn
Germany

Richard F. Spaide, MD
Professor of Ophthalmology
Vitreous, Retina Macula
Consultants of New York
460 Park Ave., 5th Floor
New York, NY 10022
USA

Dr. med. Steffen Schmitz-Valckenberg
Department of Ophthalmology
University of Bonn
Ernst-Abbe-Str. 2
53127 Bonn
Germany

Alan C. Bird, MD
Professor of
Medical Ophthalmology
Institute of Ophthalmology
University College London
11–43 Bath Street
London EC1V 9EL
United Kingdom

Library of Congress Control Number: 2007931906

ISBN   978-3-540-71993-9   Springer Berlin Heidelberg New York

Springer-Verlag is a part of Springer Science+Business Media
springer.com

Editor: Marion Philipp, Heidelberg, Germany
Desk Editor: Martina Himberger, Heidelberg, Germany
Cover design: Frido Steinen-Broo, eStudio Calamar, Spain
Typesetting and Production: LE-TEX Jelonek, Schmidt & Vöckler GbR, Leipzig, Germany

Printed on acid-free paper   24/3180/YL   5 4 3 2 1 0

Preface

It has been known for many years from histopathological studies that autofluorescence is present in the retinal pigment epithelium (RPE) due to the presence of lipofuscin. The demonstration that the excitation spectrum of the "orange-red" fluorophores extends into the visible range indicated that imaging of lipofuscin was accessible to in vivo excitation. However, in vivo recording in humans of autofluorescence using spectrophotometric techniques and imaging with a scanning laser ophthalmoscope are relatively recent.

It is believed that the level of autofluorescence represents a balance between accumulation and clearance of lipofuscin. Accumulation of fluorescent material in the RPE reflects the level of metabolic activity, which is largely determined by the quantity of photoreceptor outer segment renewal. Abnormally high levels are thought to be due to RPE cell dysfunction or to the RPE's being subjected to an abnormal metabolic load as occurs in Stargardt disease, in which the discs contain abnormally high levels of N-retinylidene-N-retinylethanolamine (A2-E). Evidence of clearance is derived from the observation that outer retinal degeneration is associated with decreased autofluorescence. This could be due to a variety of factors. There appears to be constant degradation of residual bodies in the RPE. There is evidence of photodegradation of A2-E, and in addition, long-term phagolysosomes may be discharged from the RPE cells into the extracellular space.

It is now clear that autofluorescence imaging is useful for diagnosis in patients with visual loss and that certain inherited disorders have distinctive patterns of change. Perhaps more important is the ability to assess the state of the RPE/photoreceptor complex in ageing. Until recently the only index of ageing was the state of Bruch's membrane as indicated by the number, size, and distribution of drusen. It is now possible to assess changes in the RPE, and it has been recognised for some years that the RPE plays a crucial role in the pathogenesis of age-related macular disease (AMD). It has been shown that the pattern of autofluorescence varies among patients. However, there is marked symmetry between the eyes of those with bilateral early AMD, implying that autofluorescence characteristics reflect the risk factors, whether genetic or environmental. Furthermore, it is believed that geographic atrophy is preceded by focal increases in autofluorescence, and this belief has given rise to concepts regarding pathological processes in this form of late disease. Lipofuscin is a free radical generator when illuminated with blue light. It also acts as a surfactant that causes leakage of membranes and a rise in the pH of phagolysosomes, with consequent predictable loss of activity of degradative enzymes. In turn, lack of recycling from phagosomes may result in lack of material for outer segment renewal and photoreceptor cell death. Of perhaps the greatest importance is the ability to verify the integrity of the RPE/photoreceptor complex prior to treatment of choroidal neovascularisation such that the likely therapeutic outcome may be determined. This can be verified on the basis of autofluorescence imaging. If it is shown that therapeutic benefit can be predicted by autofluorescence imaging, it should become a routine part of the management of such cases, particularly in light of the therapeutic results of the new biological agents.

The value of autofluorescence imaging to clinical practice has been shown beyond any doubt, although, as with many new techniques, the clinical value of the technique has yet to be fully understood. It gives information that is of major clinical importance but is not yet accessible by any other technique.

In this book the principles of autofluorescence imaging are explained, the scope of the technique is summarised, and its application in clinical practice is illustrated. It is hoped that this information will help make the technique more widely available and of greater value to the clinician.

London, Juli 2007
Alan C. Bird

Contents

Contributors

Almut Bindewald-Wittich, Dr. med.
Department of Ophthalmology
University of Bonn
Ernst-Abbe-Str. 2
53127 Bonn
Germany

Alan C. Bird, MD
Professor of
Medical Ophthalmology
Institute of Ophthalmology
University College London
11–43 Bath Street
London EC1V 9EL
United Kingdom

Samantha S. Dandekar, MD
Moorfields Eye Hospital
162 City Road
London EC1V 2PD
United Kingdom

François C. Delori, PhD
Senior Scientist and Associate Professor
Vision and Visual Optics
Schepens Eye Research Institute
Harvard Medical School
20 Staniford Street
Boston, MA 02114
USA

Fred W. Fitzke, PhD
Professor of Visual Science
and Psychophysics
Visual Science
Institute of Ophthalmology
University College London
11–43 Bath Street
London EC1V 9EL
United Kingdom

Monika Fleckenstein, Dr. med.
Department of Ophthalmology
University of Bonn
Ernst-Abbe-Str. 2
53127 Bonn
Germany

Hans-Martin Helb
Department of Ophthalmology
University of Bonn
Ernst-Abbe-Str. 2
53127 Bonn, Germany

Frank G. Holz, Prof. Dr. med.
Department of Ophthalmology
University of Bonn
Ernst-Abbe-Str. 2
53127 Bonn
Germany

Peter Charbel Issa, Dr. med.
Department of Ophthalmology
University of Bonn
Ernst-Abbe-Str. 2
53127 Bonn
Germany

Claudia Keilhauer, Dr. med.
Department of Ophthalmology
University Hospital
Josef-Schneider-Str. 11
97080 Würzburg
Germany

Vy Luong
Visual Science
Institute of Ophthalmology
University College London
11–43 Bath Street
London EC1V 9EL
United Kingdom

Daniel Pauleikhoff, Prof. Dr. med.
Klinik für Augenheilkunde
St. Franziskus Hospital
Hohenzollernring 74
48145 Muenster
Germany

Felix Roth, Dr. med.
Department of Ophthalmology
University of Bonn
Ernst-Abbe-Str. 2
53127 Bonn
Germany

Steffen Schmitz-Valckenberg, Dr. med.
Institute of Ophthalmology
University College London and
Department of Ophthalmology
University of Bonn
Ernst-Abbe-Str. 2
53127 Bonn
Germany

Hendrik P.N. Scholl, Priv.-Doz. Dr. med.
Department of Ophthalmology
University of Bonn
Ernst-Abbe-Str. 2
53127 Bonn
Germany

Richard F. Spaide, MD
Professor of Ophthalmology
Vitreous, Retina
Macula Consultants of New York
and Lu Esther T. Mertz Retinal Research
Center, Manhatten Eye, Ear and Throat
Hospital
460 Park Ave., 5th Floor
New York, NY 10022
USA

Janet R. Sparrow, PhD
Anthony Donn Professor
Department of Ophthalmology
Columbia University
630 W. 168th Street
New York, NY 10032

Giovanni Staurenghi, MD, Prof.
Department of Clinical Science Luigi
Sacco
University of Milan
Via GB Grassi, 74
20157 Milan
Italy

Frederik J.G.M. van Kuijk, MD, PhD
Professor of Ophthalmology
Vice Chair for Clinical Services
Department of Ophthalmology
& Visual Sciences
University of Texas Medical Branch
Galveston, TX 77555-1106
USA

Andrea von Rückmann,
Priv.-Doz. Dr. med.
Forchstrasse 138
8032 Zürich
Switzerland

Andrew R. Webster, MD
University Senior Lecturer
Institute of Ophthalmology
University College London
11-43 Bath Street
London EC1V 9EL
United Kingdom

Sebastian Wolf, Prof. Dr.-Ing. Dr. med.
Department of Ophthalmology
Inselspital
University Bern
Freiburgstrasse
3010 Bern
Switzerland

Ute E.K. Wolf-Schnurrbusch, Dr. med.
Department of Ophthalmology
Inselspital
University Bern
Freiburgstrasse
3010 Bern
Switzerland

Part I
Methodology

Lipofuscin of the Retinal Pigment Epithelium

Janet R. Sparrow

1.1
Introduction

It is well known that the major source of fundus autofluorescence (FAF) is the lipofuscin of retinal pigment epithelial (RPE) cells. Lipofuscin is understood to be material in the lysosomal compartment of nondividing cells that cannot be degraded, and thus it accumulates [16, 74, 89]. For many cell types, lipofuscin originates internally (autophagy), but for the RPE, lipofuscin derives primarily from phagocytosed photoreceptor outer segments. These fluorophores most likely accumulate in RPE cells because the structures of the fluorophores are unusual and not amenable to degradation, rather than because the lysosomal enzymes in these cells are defective. Emerging evidence indicates that the lipofuscin of RPE cells is unique, since much of this material forms as a consequence of the light-capturing function of the retina. An origin from retinoids that leave the visual cycle is consistent with the finding that the accumulation of RPE lipofuscin is most marked in central retina, the area having the greatest concentration of visual pigment. The extensive system of conjugated double bonds within these retinoid-derived fluorophores also explains the long wavelength fluorescence emission of RPE lipofuscin. The excessive accumulation of RPE lipofuscin in autosomal-recessive Stargardt macular degeneration is considered to be the cause of RPE atrophy. This material is also implicated in disease processes underlying dominant Stargardt-like macular degeneration, Best's vitelliform macular dystrophy, and age-related macular degeneration.

1.2
The Source of RPE Lipofuscin

Evidence that the precursors of RPE lipofuscin originate in photoreceptor outer segments came from work in the Royal College of Surgeons rat showing that in this strain, in which RPE cells fail to phagocytose shed outer segment membrane, RPE lipofuscin is substantially diminished [36]. Lipofuscin was also reduced concomitant with light-induced loss of photoreceptor cells [38]. As with other cell types, the lipofuscin of RPE gathers within membrane-bound organelles of the lysosomal compartment of the cells; because of their ultrastructural appearance, these organelles are referred to as lipofuscin granules [11, 15, 27, 30]. Early theories as to the genesis of RPE lipofuscin focused on the adducts generated following the peroxidation of lipid, particularly those formed by reactions between aldehyde products and biological amines [13]. Products of lipid oxidation have been detected in lipofuscin granules [62], but whether they contribute to the golden-yellow emission of RPE lipofuscin has been a matter of discussion [14, 23, 24].

Current understanding of the molecular composition of RPE lipofuscin originated with experiments documenting that the deposition of lipofuscin fluorophores is dependent on dietary vitamin A [37]. More recently it has been shown that when the 11-*cis*-retinal and all-*trans*-retinal chromophores of visual pigment are absent, as in $Rpe65^{-/-}$ mice, RPE lipofuscin, measured as fluorescence intensity, is severely reduced [39]. These findings are consistent with the observation that in patients with early-onset retinal dystrophy associated with mutations in RPE65, RPE lipofuscin is similarly lacking [45].

1.3
Characteristics of Known RPE Lipofuscin Pigments

This evidence—that the RPE lipofuscin that accumulates with age and in some retinal disorders forms largely as a byproduct of light-related vitamin A cycling—is consistent with the finding that a prominent constituent is a di-retinal conjugate A2E ($C_{42}H_{58}NO$, molecular weight 592), named because it could be synthesized from vitamin A aldehyde (all-*trans*-retinal) and ethanolamine when combined in a 2:1 ratio [26, 58] (Figs. 1.1 and 1.2). The polar head group of A2E is a pyridine ring carrying a positive charge conferred by a quaternary amine nitrogen; two side arms extend from the ring, a long arm and a short arm. Each arm is derived from a molecule of all-*trans*-retinal [58]. The structure of A2E is unprecedented.

The polyene structure of the long arm of A2E (Fig. 1.1), including the double bonds within the pyridine and ionone rings, provides the extended conjugation system that allows A2E to absorb at wavelengths in the visible range of the spectrum. Since the absorbance spectrum of A2E has two peaks, it is also clear that the two arms of A2E do not constitute a single continuous conjugation system. Instead, A2E has an absorbance maximum in the visible spectrum of ~440 nm that can be assigned to the long arm and a shorter wavelength absorbance at ~340 nm that is generated within the short arm.

The emission spectrum of in vivo FAF exhibits strong similarities with that of cell-associated A2E and with the emission spectra of native lipofuscin present in RPE isolated from human eyes (F. Delori and J.R. Sparrow, unpublished observations) and isolated lipofuscin granules [11]. All have emission maxima at 590–620 nm and exhibit a characteristic red shift with increasing excitation wavelengths (Fig. 1.3).

Conversely, the in vivo excitation spectra are broader and peak at longer wavelengths (470–500) than that of A2E (448 nm) and native lipofuscin (460–475 nm).

The biosynthesis of A2E begins in photoreceptor outer segments with condensation reactions between all-*trans*-retinal and phosphatidylethanolamine (Fig. 1.2). All-*trans*-retinal that participates in A2E biosynthesis is generated by photoisomerization of 11-*cis* retinal. N-retinylidene-PE (NRPE), the product of the Schiff-base reaction between a single all-*trans*-retinal and phosphatidylethanolamine [42, 77, 84], is likely the substrate for ABCA4 (ABCR), the photoreceptor-specific ATP-binding cassette transporter [4, 50, 51, 53, 76–79] that is the protein product of the gene responsible for recessive Stargardt disease, a majority of cases of autosomal recessive cone-rod dystrophy, and a form of autosomal recessive retinitis pigmentosa (RP19) [3, 63]. A2E formation continues with the reaction of NRPE and a second all-*trans*-retinal and then proceeds through a multistep pathway that includes the generation of a phosphatidyl-dihydropyridinium (dihydro-A2PE) compound. The latter intermediate is unstable and undergoes oxidative aromatization [6, 42, 54] to form A2PE, the phosphatidyl-pyridinium bisretinoid that is the immediate precursor to A2E [6, 42, 54]. Because the intermediates that form before dihydro-A2PE are likely capable of reverse-synthesis, auto-oxidation of dihydro-A2PE may be the last step at which it is possible to intervene in the synthesis of A2E [71]. A2PE has a stable aromatic ring and is the fluorescent pigment detected in photoreceptor outer segments [6, 42]. Since the shedding and phagocytosis of outer segment membrane leads to the complete replacement of the photoreceptor outer segment approximately every 10 days [90], A2PE is not continuously amassed by the photoreceptor cell. In Royal College of Surgeons rats, a strain in which RPE cells fail to phagocytose shed outer segment membrane, A2PE is responsible, at least in part, for a golden-yellow autofluorescence in outer-segment degenerating debris [25, 36, 42]. A2PE may also account in part for the lipofuscin-like fluorescence detectable in photoreceptor cells in recessive Stargardt disease and in some forms of retinitis pigmentosa [10, 12, 80]. Although cleavage of A2PE to generate A2E has been suggested to occur by acid hydrolysis within RPE lysosomes [6], it is just as likely that the generation of A2E from A2PE is enzyme mediated, and phospholipase D has been implicated in this process [42].

Another constituent of RPE lipofuscin is the fluorophore isoA2E (Figs. 1.1 and 1.2) that forms by photoisomerization of A2E [54]. While the double bonds along the side arms of A2E are all in the trans (E) position, the double bond at the C13–14 position of isoA2E assumes the cis (Z) configuration [54]. Other less abundant cis-isomers— Z-olefins at the C9/9'–10/10' and C11/11'–12/12' positions—are also detectable as additional components of the lipofuscin isolated from aging human RPE [6]. For isoA2E and the other photoisomers, absorbance spectra are slightly blue-shifted relative to A2E (Fig. 1.3). A2E and its isomers have been detected in isolated human RPE [54], wherein their levels have also been shown to increase with age (Jang and Sparrow, unpublished observation). These pigments have also been demonstrated within eyecups harvested from mice, with levels being increased several fold in the *Abcr* null mutant mouse, a model of recessive Stargardt macular degeneration [40, 47–49, 84].

At least two compounds in RPE lipofuscin have ~510 nm absorbance and form by pathways distinct from that of A2E [28, 29]. Studies indicate that the pigment all-*trans*-retinal dimer, phosphatidylethanolamine (atRAL dimer-PE) (Fig. 1.1), is generated after two molecules of all-*trans*-retinal condense to form an aldehyde-bearing dimer (atRAL dimer) (Fig. 1.1). By means of its aldehyde group, atRAL dimer then forms a conjugate with phosphatidylethanolamine, thus forming atRAL dimer-PE [28, 29] (Fig. 1.1). A second ~510 nm absorbing species, all-*trans*-retinal dimer-E (atRAL dimer-E) (Fig. 1.1), can be subsequently generated by phosphate cleavage of atRAL dimer-PE. The pigments atRAL dimer-PE and atRAL dimer-E are composed of two polyene arms—seven double-bond conjugations on the long arm and four on the short—extending from a cyclohexadiene ring that is linked by Schiff base to phosphatidylethanolamine or ethanolamine, respectively. These pigments exhibit an absorbance maximum in the visible spectrum that is red-shifted relative to A2E (A2E/isoA2E, λ_{max} ~340, 440 nm; atRAL dimer-PE, λ_{max} ~290, 510 nm). The relatively long wavelength absorbance of atRAL dimer-PE and atRAL dimer-E is attributable to protonation of the Schiff base linkage in these compounds. The fluorescence emission of these pigments peaks at approximately 600 nm and is relatively weak in intensity (Fig. 1.3). It is also significant that when deprotonated, these pigments undergo hydrolysis to revert to atRAL dimer. Unprotonated/unconjugated atRAL dimer is detected in mice and human eyes along with conjugated/protonated atRAL dimer-PE and atRAL dimer-E, indicating that in the acidic environment in which these pigments are housed (lysosomal compartment), an equilibrium exists between the deprotonated/unconjugated and protonated/conjugated states. The absorbance

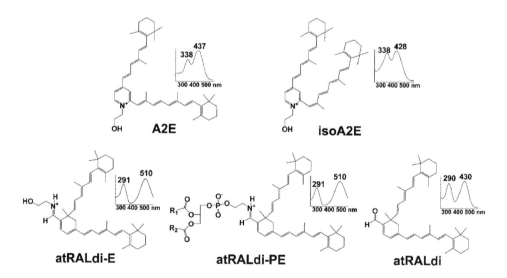

Fig. 1.1 Structures of retinal pigment epithelial (RPE) lipofuscin pigments A2E, isoA2E, all-*trans*-retinal dimer-ethanolamine (atRALdi-E), all-*trans*-retinal dimer-phosphatidylethanolamine (atRALdi-PE), and all-*trans*-retinal dimer (atRALdi) with corresponding ultraviolet-visible absorbance spectra

spectrum of unconjugated atRAL dimer exhibits maxima at ~290 and 432 nm, and its fluorescence emission profile (emission maximum 580 nm with 430 nm excitation) is slightly different from that of A2E (Fig. 1.3). The pigments atRAL dimer-PE and atRAL dimer-E are present at elevated levels in the lipofuscin-filled RPE of *Abcr* null mutant mice (S. Kim and J.R. Sparrow, unpublished).

Additional components of RPE lipofuscin are generated by photooxidation. In the case of A2E, photooxidation was originally suspected because of the fluorescence bleaching that accompanies irradiation. Subsequent analysis by mass spectrometry revealed that following blue light irradiation of A2E, the profile not only consisted of the M+ 592 peak attributable to A2E but also included a series of peaks, the sizes of which increased by increments of mass 16, indicating the addition of oxygens at carbon–carbon double bonds [5, 70].

The mixture of oxygen-containing moieties within photooxidized A2E includes cyclic peroxides (peroxy-A2E), furanoid oxides (furano-A2E), and probably epoxides [5, 21, 35]. We have also shown that oxidation occurs more readily on the short arm of A2E. Intracellular A2E has been shown to undergo photooxidation upon blue-

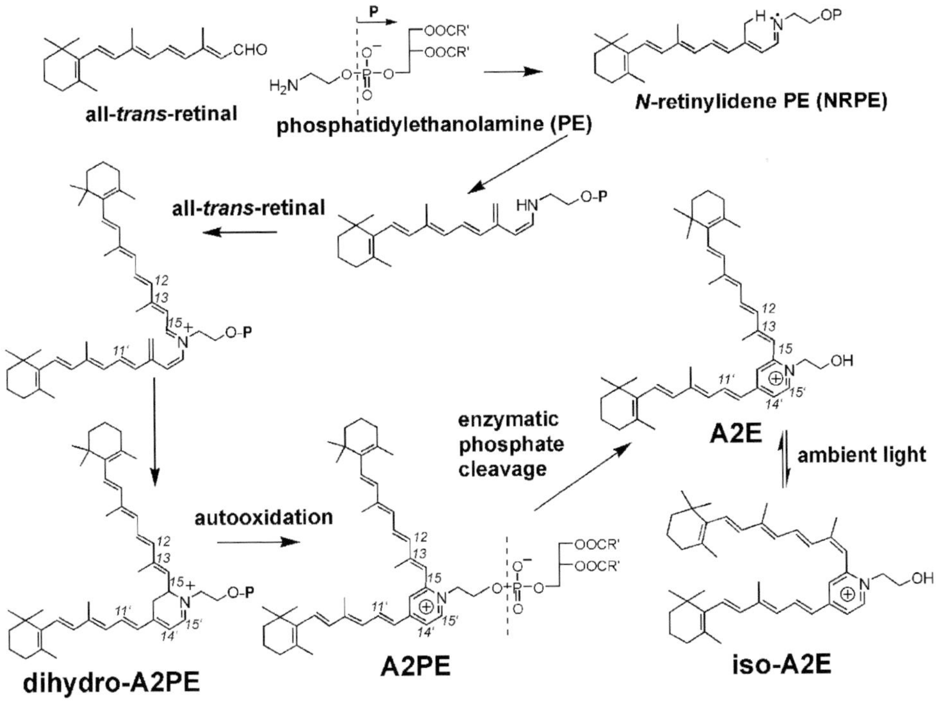

Fig. 1.2 Biosynthesis pathway of A2E and the photoisomer isoA2E from all-*trans*-retinal and phosphatidylethanolamine. The immediate precursor A2PE forms in outer segments; phosphate hydrolysis of A2PE to generate A2E and isoA2E probably occurs in retinal pigment epithelial lysosomes via an enzyme-mediated mechanism

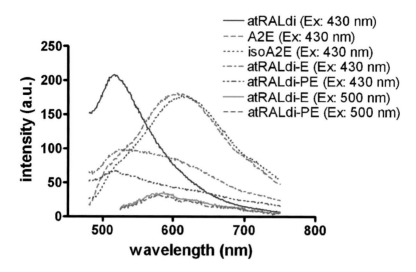

Fig. 1.3 Emission spectra of A2E, isoA2E, all-*trans*-retinal dimer-ethanolamine (atRALdi-E), all-*trans*-retinal dimer-phosphatidylethanolamine (atRALdi-PE), and all-*trans*-retinal dimer (atRALdi) with excitation at 430 or 500 nm, as indicated

light exposure [70], and we have detected monofuran-A2E and monoperoxy-A2E in RPE from human eyes and in eyecups from mice with null mutations in *Abcr*[-/-] [35], the gene responsible for recessive Stargardt disease. Since the cytotoxicity of oxygen-containing groups such as endoperoxides is well known [46, 81], these moieties may account, at least in part, for cellular damage ensuing from A2E accumulation [73]. The addition of oxygens at olefins of A2E is associated with blue shifts in absorbance. For instance, when one furan or peroxy moiety is positioned on the long arm of A2E, the long wavelength absorbance changes to ~402 nm. Although monoperoxy-A2E exhibits a fluorescence emission that is more intense than A2E, with further oxidation, autofluorescence diminishes.

1.4
Adverse Effects of RPE Lipofuscin

In autosomal-recessive Stargardt disease caused by *ABCA4/ABCR* gene mutations [2, 64, 65, 88], RPE lipofuscin has a composition similar to age-associated lipofuscin; the accumulation of this material is also accelerated [19, 22, 43, 44, 82] and is considered the cause of RPE atrophy [56]. Since RPE lipofuscin is amassed with age and is of highest concentration underlying central retina [20], it is also implicated in atrophic age-related macular degeneration. Additionally, in-vivo monitoring of RPE lipofuscin as FAF in patients with age-related macular degeneration has revealed areas of intense FAF that correspond to sites of reduced scotopic sensitivity [59, 60] and are prone to atrophy [31, 33]. Because mutations in *ABCA4/ABCR* lead to increased RPE lipofuscin, it is also of interest that heterozygous mutations in the gene have been associated with increased susceptibility to age-related macular degeneration [2, 9]. Poorly understood is the relationship between RPE lipofuscin and vitelliform macular dystrophies (e.g., Best disease, adult-onset vitelliform dystrophy) caused by mutations in VMD2, the gene encoding bestrophin-1 (Best1).

Work in in-vitro models suggests mechanisms by which lipofuscin constituents may damage the RPE cell [18, 61, 67, 68, 75]. Thus, as an amphiphilic molecule, not only can A2E mediate detergent-like effects on cell membranes [18, 67, 72, 75], but its accumulation can lead to the alkalinization of lysosomes [32], possibly by interfering with the ATPase-dependent proton pump located in the lysosomal membrane [7]. A2E appears not to directly inhibit the activities of lysosomal enzymes [8]. A2E has also been shown to confer a susceptibility to photo-induced apoptosis [61, 68, 69], with sensitivity to blue light being directly dependent on the A2E content of the cells; green light (540 nm) is considerably less damaging. The photochemical events triggering apoptosis when A2E-laden RPE are exposed to blue light probably involve the generation of reactive forms of oxygen and photooxidative products of A2E (discussed above). The amount of A2E that undergoes photooxidation and cleavage in a lifetime may be significant: we observed that the amount of formed A2-PE, the immediate precursor of A2E, is many times greater than the amounts of A2E that accumulate in RPE cells [41]. One explanation for this finding is that a portion of the A2E that forms is normally lost. Because it is known that levels of A2E in RPE do not diminish under dark conditions [48], it is likely that the light-dependent conditions involve photooxidative processes. Decreased FAF is observed in areas of photoreceptor cell degeneration [83]; perhaps this observation can be accounted for by halted deposition (due to the absence of photoreceptor cells) together with depletion due to photooxidation.

1.5
Modulators of RPE Lipofuscin Formation

All-*trans*-retinal that avoids reduction to all-*trans*-retinol by all-*trans*-retinol dehydrogenase is available to undergo the random inadvertent reactions that lead to formation of the all-*trans*-retinal-derived fluorophores of RPE lipofuscin. Correspondingly, conditions that increase the availability of all-*trans*-retinal enhance the opportunity for these fluorophores to form. Not surprisingly, therefore, since the generation of all-*trans*-retinal in photoreceptor outer segments is light-dependent, light is also a determinant of the rate of A2E formation. Thus, in-vivo experiments have shown that the A2E precursor A2PE in photoreceptor outer segments is augmented by exposing rats to bright light [6]. Moreover, dark rearing of ABCR$^{-/-}$ mice inhibits the deposition of A2E [48]. Since A2E levels are not diminished if mice are raised in cyclic light and then transferred to darkness, it is also clear that once A2E is formed, it is not eliminated from the RPE [48]. Another well-known factor that modulates

A2E formation is the activity of ABCA4 (ABCR), the photoreceptor-specific ATP-binding cassette transporter [50, 53, 76, 79] that is thought to aid in the movement of all-*trans*-retinal to the cytosolic side of the disc membrane [1, 34, 76, 79, 84], where it is accessible to retinol dehydrogenase, the enzyme responsible for its reduction to all-*trans*-retinol [57]. As a consequence of the loss of ABCR protein activity in *Abcr*[-/-] mice, the levels of A2E in RPE cells are several fold greater than those in normal mice [40, 47, 84]. In *Abcr*[+/-] mice, accumulation of A2E is approximately 40% of that in the null mutant mouse [49].

Because the source of all-*trans*-retinal for A2E formation is the photoisomerization of 11-*cis*-retinal, another determinant of A2E accumulation is the kinetics of 11-*cis*-retinal regeneration. Evidence for this factor has come from studies of an amino acid variant in murine Rpe65, the visual cycle protein that may have a rate-determining role in the visual cycle [87]. Specifically, in albino and pigmented mice in which the amino acid residue at position 450 of RPE 65 is methionine (C57BL/6J-c[2J]; *Abcr*[-/-] Met/Met; *Abcr*[+/+] Met/Met) instead of leucine (BALB/cByJ; *Abcr*[-/-] Leu/Leu; *Abcr*[+/+] Leu/Leu), recovery of the electroretinographic response following a photobleach and rhodopsin regeneration are retarded [17, 52, 85, 86]; the content of A2E in the RPE is diminished by a similar magnitude [40].

Therapeutic approaches aimed at retarding the visual cycle also serve to reduce A2E accumulation. For instance, the acne medication isotretinoin (13-*cis*-retinoic acid, Accutane; Roche Laboratories, Nutley, NJ), which was shown to reduce visual sensitivity under darkened conditions by retarding 11-*cis*-retinal regeneration [66], reduces A2E deposition in the RPE of ABCR[-/-] mice [55]. Nonetheless, 13-*cis*-retinoic acid has severe side effects, including teratogenicity [71] and is thus not appropriate for long-term therapy. Nonretinoid isoprenoid compounds that compete with retinyl esters for binding to RPE65, thereby interfering with visual cycle kinetics [47], also serve to mediate substantial reductions in A2E accumulation when administered chronically to *Abcr*[-/-] mice. Indeed, RPE65 appears to be an excellent therapeutic target, with A2E levels in eyecups of *Abcr*[-/-] mice treated with the RPE65 antagonists being as much as 85% lower than in vehicle-treated mice [47]. In another form of intervention, A2E levels in *Abcr*[-/-] mice have also been reduced by daily administration of the retinoic acid analog N-(4-hydroxyphenyl)retinamide (HPR) for 1 month [56]. HPR acts by competing for binding sites on retinol-binding protein, thus reducing serum retinol levels. Consequently, retinol uptake by the eye is reduced, visual cycle retinoids are decreased, and the associated decrease in all-*trans*-retinal leads to retarded A2E formation.

1.6
Summary

RPE cells are unusual in that they are exposed to visible light while at the same time housing photoreactive molecules that accumulate as lipofuscin. There are many indications that an excessive accumulation of RPE lipofuscin can lead to cellular dysfunction and contribute to retinal aging and degeneration [74]. Insight into the composition, biogenesis, and photoreactivity of RPE lipofuscin has improved our understanding of the extent to which the accumulation of these pigments renders the macula prone to insult. Novel therapeutic approaches are being developed to minimize lipofuscin accumulation in order to reduce the progression of retinal conditions such as recessive Stargardt disease and age-related macular degeneration.

Acknowledgements

Supported by the National Eye Institute (EY 12951), the Foundation Fighting Blindness, the Steinbach Fund, and unrestricted funds to the Department of Ophthalmology, Columbia University, from Research to Prevent Blindness. JRS is a recipient of an Alcon Research Institute Award.

References

1. Ahn J, Wong JT, Molday RS (2000) The effect of lipid environment and retinoids on the ATPase activity of ABCR, the photoreceptor ABC transporter responsible for Stargardt macular dystrophy. J Biol Chem 275:20399–20405

2. Allikmets R, Shroyer NF, Singh N, Seddon JM, Lewis RA, Bernstein PS, Peiffer A, Zabriskie NA, Li Y, Hutchinson A, Dean M, Lupski JR, Leppert M (1997) Mutation of the Stargardt disease gene (ABCR) in age-related macular degeneration. Science 277:1805–1807

3. Allikmets R, Singh N, Sun H, Shroyer NF, Hutchinson A, Chidambaram A, Gerrard B, Baird L, Stauffer D, Peiffer A, Rattner A, Smallwood P, Li Y, Anderson KL, Lewis RA, Nathans J, Leppert M, Dean M, Lupski JR (1997) A photoreceptor cell-specific ATP-binding transporter gene (ABCR) is mutated in recessive Stargardt macular dystrophy. Nat Genet 15:236–246

4. Beharry S, Zhong M, Molday RS (2004) N-retinylidene-phosphatidylethanolamine is the preferred retinoid substrate for the photoreceptor-specific ABC transporter ABCA4 (ABCR). J Biol Chem 279:53972–53979

5. Ben-Shabat S, Itagaki Y, Jockusch S, Sparrow JR, Turro NJ, Nakanishi K (2002) Formation of a nona-oxirane from A2E, a lipofuscin fluorophore related to macular degeneration, and evidence of singlet oxygen involvement. Angew Chem Int Ed 41:814–817

6. Ben-Shabat S, Parish CA, Vollmer HR, Itagaki Y, Fishkin N, Nakanishi K, Sparrow JR (2002) Biosynthetic studies of A2E, a major fluorophore of RPE lipofuscin. J Biol Chem 277:7183–7190

7. Bergmann M, Schutt F, Holz FG, Kopitz J (2004) Inhibition of the ATP-driven proton pump in RPE lysosomes by the major lipofuscin fluorophore A2-E may contribute to the pathogenesis of age-related macular degeneration. FASEB J 18:562–564

8. Berman M, Schutt F, Holz FG, Kopitz J (2001) Does A2E, a retinoid component of lipofuscin and inhibitor of lysosomal degradative functions, directly affect the activity of lysosomal hydrolases. Exp Eye Res 72:191–195

9. Bernstein PS, Leppert M, Singh N, Dean M, Lewis RA, Lupski JR, Allikmets R, Seddon JM (2002) Genotype-phenotype analysis of ABCR variants in macular degeneration probands and siblings. Invest Ophthalmol Vis Sci 43:466–473

10. Birnbach CD, Jarvelainen M, Possin DE, Milam AH (1994) Histopathology and immunocyto-chemistry of the neurosensory retina in fundus flavimaculatus. Ophthalmology 101:1211–1219

11. Boulton M, Docchio F, Dayhaw-Barker P, Ramponi R, Cubeddu R (1990) Age-related changes in the morphology, absorption and fluorescence of melanosomes and lipofuscin granules of the retinal pigment epithelium. Vision Res 30:1291–1303

12. Bunt-Milam AH, Kalina RE, Pagon RA (1983) Clinical-ultrastructural study of a retinal dys-trophy. Invest Ophthalmol Vis Sci 24:458–469

13. Chio KS, Reiss U, Fletcher B, Tappel AL (1969) Peroxidation of subcellular organelles: for-mation of lipofuscin-like fluorescent pigments. Science 166:1535–1536

14. Chowdhury PK, Halder M, Choudhury PK, Kraus GA, Desai MJ, Armstrong DW, Casey TA, Rasmussen MA, Petrich JW (2004) Generation of fluorescent adducts of malondialdehyde and amino acids: toward an understanding of lipofuscin. Photochem Photobiol 79:21–25

15. Clancy CMR, Krogmeier JR, Pawlak A, Rozanowska M, Sarna T, Dunn RC, Simon JD (2000) Atomic force microscopy and near-field scanning optical microscopy measurements of sin-gle human retinal lipofuscin granules. J Phys Chem B 104:12098–12101

16. Cuervo AM, Dice JR (2000) When lysosomes get old. Exp Gerontol 35:119–131

17. Danciger M, Matthes MT, Yasamura D, Akhmedov NB, Rickabaugh T, Gentleman S, Red-mond TM, La Vail MM, Farber DB (2000) A QTL on distal chromosome 3 that influences the severity of light-induced damage to mouse photoreceptors. Mam Genome 11:422–427

18. De S, Sakmar TP (2002) Interaction of A2E with model membranes. Implications to the pathogenesis of age-related macular degeneration. J Gen Physiol 120:147–157

19. Delori FC, Staurenghi G, Arend O, Dorey CK, Goger DG, Weiter JJ (1995) In vivo measure-ment of lipofuscin in Stargardt's disease–Fundus flavimaculatus. Invest Ophthalmol Vis Sci 36:2327–2331

20. Delori FC, Goger DG, Dorey CK (2001) Age-related accumulation and spatial distribution of lipofuscin in RPE of normal subjects. Invest Ophthalmol Vis Sci 42:1855–1866

21. Dillon J, Wang Z, Avalle LB, Gaillard ER (2004) The photochemical oxidation of A2E results in the formation of a 5,8,5',8'-bis-furanoid oxide. Exp Eye Res 79:537–542

22. Eagle RC, Lucier AC, Bernardino VB, Yanoff M (1980) Retinal pigment epithelial abnormal-ities in fundus flavimaculatus. Ophthalmol 87:1189–1200

23. Eldred G, Katz ML (1991) The lipid peroxidation theory of lipofuscinogenesis cannot yet be confirmed. Free Rad Biol Med 10:445–447

24. Eldred GE, Katz ML (1989) The autofluorescent products of lipid peroxidation may not be lipofuscin-like [see comments]. Free Radic Biol Med 7:157–163

25. Eldred GE (1991) The fluorophores of the RCS rat retina and implications for retinal degen-eration. CRC Press, Boca Raton, Florida

26. Eldred GE, Lasky MR (1993) Retinal age pigments generated by self-assembling lysosomo-tropic detergents. Nature 361:724–726

27. Feeney-Burns L, Eldred GE (1983) The fate of the phagosome: conversion to "age pigment" and impact in human retinal pigment epithelium. Trans Ophthalmol Soc UK 103:416–421

28. Fishkin N, Pescitelli G, Sparrow JR, Nakanishi K, Berova N (2004) Absolute configurational determination of an all-trans-retinal dimer isolated from photoreceptor outer segments. Chirality 16:637–641

29. Fishkin NE, Pescitelli G, Itagaki Y, Berova N, Allikmets R, Nakanishi K, Sparrow JR (2004) Isolation and characterization of a novel RPE cell fluorophore: all-trans-retinal dimer conjugate. Invest Ophthalmol Vis Sci 45:E–abstract 1803

30. Haralampus-Grynaviski NM, Lamb LE, Clancy CMR, Skumatz C, Burke JM, Sarna T, Simon JD (2003) Spectroscopic and morphological studies of human retinal lipofuscin granules. Proc Natl Acad Sci USA 100:3179–3184

31. Holz FG, Bellmann C, Margaritidis M, Schutt F, Otto TP, Volcker HE (1999) Patterns of increased in vivo fundus autofluorescence in the junctional zone of geographic atrophy of the retinal pigment epithelium associated with age-related macular degeneration. Graefe's Arch Clin Exp Ophthalmol 237:145–152

32. Holz FG, Schutt F, Kopitz J, Eldred GE, Kruse FE, Volcker HE, Cantz M (1999) Inhibition of lysosomal degradative functions in RPE cells by a retinoid component of lipofuscin. Invest Ophthalmol Vis Sci 40:737–743

33. Holz FG, Bellman C, Staudt S, Schutt F, Volcker HE (2001) Fundus autofluorescence and development of geographic atrophy in age-related macular degeneration. Invest Ophthalmol Vis Sci 42:1051–1056

34. Illing M, Molday LL, Molday RS (1997) The 220-kDa rim protein of retinal rod outer segments is a member of the ABC transporter superfamily. J Biol Chem 272:10303–10310

35. Jang YP, Matsuda H, Itagaki Y, Nakanishi K, Sparrow JR (2006) Characterization of peroxy-A2E and furan-A2E photooxidation products and detection in human and mouse retinal pigment epithelial cells lipofuscin. J Biol Chem 280:39732–39739

36. Katz ML, Drea CM, Eldred GE, Hess HH, Robison WG, Jr. (1986) Influence of early photoreceptor degeneration on lipofuscin in the retinal pigment epithelium. Exp Eye Res 43:561–573

37. Katz ML, Drea CM, Robison WG, Jr. (1986) Relationship between dietary retinol and lipofuscin in the retinal pigment epithelium. Mech Ageing Dev 35:291–305

38. Katz ML, Eldred GE (1989) Retinal light damage reduces autofluorescent pigment deposition in the retinal pigment epithelium. Invest Ophthalmol Vis Sci 30:37–43

39. Katz ML, Redmond TM (2001) Effect of Rpe65 knockout on accumulation of lipofuscin fluorophores in the retinal pigment epithelium. Invest Ophthalmol Vis Sci 42:3023–3030

40. Kim SR, Fishkin N, Kong J, Nakanishi K, Allikmets R, Sparrow JR (2004) The Rpe65 Leu-450Met variant is associated with reduced levels of the RPE lipofuscin fluorophores A2E and iso-A2E. Proc Natl Acad Sci USA 101:11668–11672

41. Kim SR, Nakanishi K, Itagaki Y, Sparrow JR (2006) Photooxidation of A2-PE, a photoreceptor outer segment fluorophore, and protection by lutein and zeaxanthin. Exp Eye Res 82:828–839

42. Liu J, Itagaki Y, Ben-Shabat S, Nakanishi K, Sparrow JR (2000) The biosynthesis of A2E, a fluorophore of aging retina, involves the formation of the precursor, A2-PE, in the photoreceptor outer segment membrane. J Biol Chem 275:29354–29360

43. Lois N, Holder GE, Fitzke FW, Plant C, Bird AC (1999) Intrafamilial variation of phenotype in Stargardt macular dystrophy-fundus flavimaculatus. Invest Ophthalmol Vis Sci 40:2668–2675

44. Lopez PF, Maumenee IH, de la Cruz Z, Green WR (1990) Autosomal-dominant fundus favimaculatus. Clinicopathologic correlation. Ophthalmol 97:798–809

45. Lorenz B, Wabbels B, Wegscheider E, Hamel CP, Drexler W, Presing MN (2004) Lack of fundus autofluorescence to 488 nanometers from childhood on in patients with early-onset severe retinal dystrophy associated with mutations in RPE65. Ophthalmol 111:1585–1594

46. Maggs JL, Bishop LPD, Batty KT, Dodd CC, Ilett KF, O'Neill PM, Edwards G, Park BK (2004) Hepatocellular bioactivation and cytotoxicity of the synthetic endoperoxide antimalarial arteflene. Chem-Biol Interact 147:173–184

47. Maiti P, Kong J, Kim SR, Sparrow JR, Allikmets R, Rando RR (2006) Small molecule RPE65 antagonists limit the visual cycle and prevent lipofuscin formation. Biochem 45:852–860

48. Mata NL, Weng J, Travis GH (2000) Biosynthesis of a major lipofuscin fluorophore in mice and humans with ABCR-mediated retinal and macular degeneration. Proc Natl Acad Sci USA 97:7154–7159

49. Mata NL, Tzekov RT, Liu X, Weng J, Birch DG, Travis GH (2001) Delayed dark adaptation and lipofuscin accumulation in abcr+/- mice: implications for involvement of ABCR in age-related macular degeneration. Invest Ophthalmol Vis Sci 42:1685–1690

50. Molday LL, Rabin AR, Molday RS (2000) ABCR expression in foveal cone photoreceptors and its role in Stargardt macular dystrophy. Nat Genet 25:257–258

51. Molday RS, Molday LL (1979) Identification and characterization of multiple forms of rhodopsin and minor proteins in frog and bovine outer segment disc membranes. Electrophoresis, lectin labeling and proteolysis studies. J Biol Chem 254:4653–4660

52. Nusinowitz S, Nguyen L, Radu RA, Kashani Z, Farber DB, Danciger M (2003) Electroretinographic evidence for altered phototransduction gain and slowed recovery from photobleaches in albino mice with a MET450 variant in RPE6. Exp Eye Res 77:627–638

53. Papermaster DS, Schneider BG, Zorn MA, Kraehenbuhl JP (1978) Immunocytochemical localization of a large intrinsic membrane protein to the incisures and margins of frog rod outer segment disks. J Cell Biol 78:415–425

54. Parish CA, Hashimoto M, Nakanishi K, Dillon J, Sparrow JR (1998) Isolation and one-step preparation of A2E and iso-A2E, fluorophores from human retinal pigment epithelium. Proc Natl Acad Sci USA 95:14609–14613

55. Radu RA, Mata NL, Nusinowitz S, Liu X, Sieving PA, Travis GH (2003) Treatment with isotretinoin inhibits lipofuscin and A2E accumulation in a mouse model of recessive Stargardt's macular degeneration. Proc Natl Acad Sci U S A 100:4742–4747

56. Radu RA, Han Y, Bui TV, Nusinowitz S, Bok D, Lichter J, Widder K, Travis GH, Mata NL (2005) Reductions in serum vitamin A arrest accumulation of toxic retinal fluorophores: a potential therapy for treatment of lipofuscin-based retinal diseases. Invest Ophthalmol Vis Sci 46:4393–4401

57. Saari JC, Garwin GG, Van Hooser JP, Palczewski K (1998) Reduction of all-trans-retinal limits regeneration of visual pigment in mice. Vision Res 38:1325–1333

58. Sakai N, Decatur J, Nakanishi K, Eldred GE (1996) Ocular age pigment "A2E": an unprecedented pyridinium bisretinoid. J Am Chem Soc 118:1559–1560

59. Schmitz-Valckenberg S, Bultmann S, Dreyhaupt J, Bindewald A, Holz FG, Rohrschneider K (2004) Fundus autofluorescence and fundus perimetry in the junctional zone of geographic atrophy in patients with age-related macular degeneration. Invest Ophthalmol Vis Sci 45:4470–4476

60. Scholl HPN, Bellmann C, Dandekar SS, Bird AC, Fitzke FW (2004) Photopic and scotopic fine matrix mapping of retinal areas of increased fundus autofluorescence in patients with age-related maculopathy. Invest Ophthalmol Vis Sci 45:574–583

61. Schutt F, Davies S, Kopitz J, Holz FG, Boulton ME (2000) Photodamage to human RPE cells by A2-E, a retinoid component of lipofuscin. Invest Ophthalmol Vis Sci 41:2303–2308

62. Schutt F, Bergmann M, Holz FG, Kopitz J (2003) Proteins modified by malondialdehyde, 4-hydroxynonenal or advanced glycation end products in lipofuscin of human retinal pigment epithelium. Invest Ophthalmol Vis Sci 44:3663–3668

63. Shroyer NF, Lewis RA, Allikmets R, Singh N, Dean M, Leppert M, Lupski JR (1999) The rod photoreceptor ATP-binding cassette transporter gene, ABCR, and retinal disease: from monogenic to multifactorial. Vision Res 39:2537–2544

64. Shroyer NF, Lewis RA, Yatsenko AN, Lupski JR (2001) Null missense ABCR (ABCA4) mutations in a family with Stargardt disease and retinitis pigmentosa. Invest Ophthalmol Vis Sci 42:2757–2761

65. Shroyer NF, Lewis RA, Yatsenko AN, Wensel TG, Lupski JR (2001) Cosegregation and functional analysis of mutant ABCR (ABCA4) alleles in families that manifest both Stargardt disease and age-related macular degeneration. Hum Mol Genet 10:2671–2678

66. Sieving PA, Chaudhry P, Kondo M, Provenzano M, Wu D, Carlson TJ, Bush RA, Thompson DA (2001) Inhibition of the visual cycle in vivo by 13-cis retinoic acid protects from light damage and provides a mechanism for night blindness in isotretinoin therapy. Proc Natl Acad Sci USA 98:1835–1840

67. Sparrow JR, Parish CA, Hashimoto M, Nakanishi K (1999) A2E, a lipofuscin fluorophore, in human retinal pigmented epithelial cells in culture. Invest Ophthalmol Vis Sci 40:2988–2995

68. Sparrow JR, Nakanishi K, Parish CA (2000) The lipofuscin fluorophore A2E mediates blue light-induced damage to retinal pigmented epithelial cells. Invest Ophthalmol Vis Sci 41:1981–1989

69. Sparrow JR, Cai B (2001) Blue light-induced apoptosis of A2E-containing RPE: involvement of caspase-3 and protection by Bcl-2. Invest Ophthalmol Vis Sci 42:1356–1362

70. Sparrow JR, Zhou J, Ben-Shabat S, Vollmer H, Itagaki Y, Nakanishi K (2002) Involvement of oxidative mechanisms in blue light induced damage to A2E-laden RPE. Invest Ophthalmol Vis Sci 43:1222–1227

71. Sparrow JR (2003) Therapy for macular degeneration: insignts from acne. Proc Natl Acad Sci USA 100:4353–4354

72. Sparrow JR, Fishkin N, Zhou J, Cai B, Jang YP, Krane S, Itagaki Y, Nakanishi K (2003) A2E, a byproduct of the visual cycle. Vision Res 43:2983–2990

73. Sparrow JR, Vollmer-Snarr HR, Zhou J, Jang YP, Jockusch S, Itagaki Y, Nakanishi K (2003) A2E-epoxides damage DNA in retinal pigment epithelial cells. Vitamin E and other antioxidants inhibit A2E-epoxide formation. J Biol Chem 278:18207–18213

74. Sparrow JR, Boulton M (2005) RPE lipofuscin and its role in retinal photobiology. Exp Eye Res 80:595–606

75. Sparrow JR, Cai B, Jang YP, Zhou J, Nakanishi K (2006) A2E, a fluorophore of RPE lipofuscin, can destabilize membrane. Adv Exp Med and Biol 572:63–68

76. Sun H, Nathans J (1997) Stargardt's ABCR is localized to the disc membrane of retinal rod outer segments. Nat Genet 17:15–16

77. Sun H, Molday RS, Nathans J (1999) Retinal stimulates ATP hydrolysis by purified and reconstituted ABCR, the photoreceptor-specific ATP-binding cassette transporter responsible for Stargardt disease. J Biol Chem 274:8269–8281

78. Sun H, Nathans J (2001) Mechanistic studies of ABCR, the ABC transporter in photoreceptor outer segments responsible for autosomal recessive Stargardt disease. J Bioenerg Biomembrane 33:523–530

79. Sun H, Nathans J (2001) ABCR, the ATP-binding cassette transporter responsible for Stargardt macular dystrophy, is an efficient target of all-trans retinal-mediated photo-oxidative damage in vitro:implications for retinal disease. J Biol Chem 276:11766–11774

80. Szamier RB, Berson EL (1977) Retinal ultrastructure in advanced retinitis pigmentosa. Invest Ophthalmol Vis Sci 16:947–962

81. Takada N, Watanabe M, Yamada A, Suenaga K, Yamada K, Ueda K, Uemura D (2001) Isolation and structures of haterumadioxins A and B, cytotoxic endoperoxides from the Okinawan Sponge Plakortis lita. J Nat Prod 64:356–359

82. von Ruckmann A, Fitzke FW, Bird AC (1997) In vivo fundus autofluorescence in macular dystrophies. Arch Ophthalmol 115:609–615

83. Von Ruckmann A, Fitzke FW, Fan J, Halfyard A, Bird AC (2002) Abnormalities of fundus autofluorescence in central serous retinopathy. Am J Ophthalmol 133:780–786

84. Weng J, Mata NL, Azarian SM, Tzekov RT, Birch DG, Travis GH (1999) Insights into the function of Rim protein in photoreceptors and etiology of Stargardt's disease from the phenotype in abcr knockout mice. Cell 98:13–23

85. Wenzel A, Reme CE, Williams TP, Hafezi F, Grimm C (2001) The Rpe65 Leu450Met variation increases retinal resistance against light-induced degeneration by slowing rhodopsin regeneration. J Neurosci 21:53–58

86. Wenzel A, Grimm C, Samardzija M, Reme CE (2003) The genetic modified Rpe65Leu$_{450}$: effect on light damage susceptibility in c-Fos-deficient mice. Invest Ophthalmol Vis Sci 44:2798–2802

87. Xue L, Gollapalli DR, Maiti P, Jahng WJ, Rando RR (2004) A palmitoylation switch mechanism in the regulation of the visual cycle. Cell 117:761–771

88. Yatsenko AN, Shroyer NF, Lewis RA, Lupski JR (2001) Late-onset Stargardt disease is associated with missense mutations that map outside known functional regions of ABCR (ABCA4). Hum Genet 108:346–355

89. Yin D (1996) Biochemical basis of lipofuscin, ceroid, and age pigment-like fluorophores. Free Rad Biol Med 21:871–888

90. Young RW (1971) The renewal of rod and cone outer segments in the rhesus monkey. J Cell Biol 49:303–318

Origin of Fundus Autofluorescence

François Delori, Claudia Keilhauer,
Janet R. Sparrow, Giovanni Staurenghi

2

2.1
Introduction

One of the important roles of the retinal pigment epithelium (RPE) is to digest, by lysosomal action, the tips of the outer segments of the photoreceptors that are phagocytosed on a daily basis. The digestion process of these materials, which contain polysaturated fatty acids and byproducts of the visual cycle, is overall very efficient, but a tiny fraction is chemically incompatible for degradation and therefore accumulates in lysosomes of the RPE. This undigested fraction is lipofuscin (LF). Over age 70, as much as 20–33% of the free cytoplasmic space of the RPE cell may be occupied by granules of LF and melanolipofuscin, a compound product of LF and melanin [1].

Potentially noxious effects of LF and A2E, one of the LF components, are discussed in Chap. 1. These effects range from photochemical blue light damage [2], inhibition of lysosomal digestion of proteins [3, 4], detergent-like disruption of membranes [5, 6], RPE apoptosis [7], and DNA damage [8, 9].

Although still controversial, it is possible that excessive levels of LF compromise essential RPE functions and contribute to the pathogenesis of age-related macular degeneration (AMD). The association between LF accumulation and retinal degeneration is most clearly delineated in Stargardt's macular dystrophy, a retinal degeneration characterized by high levels of LF [10–12] and caused by defects in the ABCA4 gene [13, 14]. Excessive LF accumulation has been described in mice carrying null mutations in the ABCR gene [15, 16]. Furthermore, loss of visual function in Best's disease [17] and Batten's disease [18] has also been attributed to excessive accumulation of LF-like materials in the lysosomes of the RPE.

Lipofuscin is a pigment that exhibits a characteristic autofluorescence when excited in ultraviolet (UV) or blue light. Fluorescence microscopy of the RPE using UV or blue excitation light reveals distinctly bright orange-red or golden-yellow granules. This fluorescence is also what makes it possible to visualize and measure LF noninvasively; the absorption spectrum of LF is monotonic without any distinct spectral signature, and it would be very challenging to measure it by reflectometry.

2.2
Spectrofluorometry of Fundus Autofluorescence (FAF)

The first in-vivo demonstration of fundus autofluorescence (FAF) came from vitreous fluorophotometry by the detection, in the pre-injection scans, of a distinct "retinal" peak whose magnitude increased with age as would be expected from LF fluorescence [19, 20]. These observations led to the development of a fundus spectrofluorometer [21, 22] specifically designed to measure the excitation and emission spectra of the autofluorescence from small retinal areas (2° diameter) of the fundus and to allow absolute measurements of the fluorescence. The device incorporated an image-intensifier diode array as detector, beam separation in the pupil, and confocal detection to minimize the contribution of autofluorescence from the crystalline lens. This device was initially used to demonstrate that LF was the dominant source of fluorescence in FAF, based on its spatial distribution, spectral characteristics, and age relationship [23].

2.3
Imaging of FAF

The autofluorescence intensity of fundus is about two orders of magnitude lower than the background of a fluorescein angiogram at the most intense part of the dye transit.

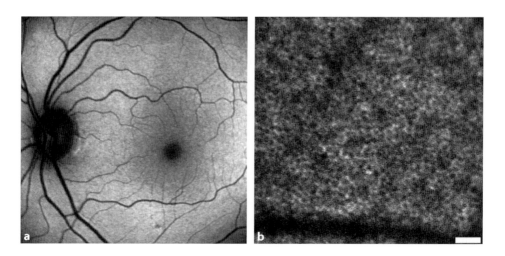

Fig. 2.1 **a** Autofluorescence images of a 55-year-old subject with normal retinal status obtained with a confocal scanning laser ophthalmoscope (SLO) and 488 nm excitation (HRAc, Heidelberg Engineering). **b** Autofluorescence image 10° superior to the fovea of a 25-year-old subject (normal retinal status), showing individual retinal pigment epithelium (RPE) cells. The image was obtained noninvasively with an adaptive optics SLO and 568 nm excitation [32]. The RPE cell nuclei appear dark and surrounded by the autofluorescent signal from lipofuscin located in the cytoplasm of the cell. (Scale bar: 50 µm) Image courtesy of Jessica I.W. Morgan and David R. Williams, University of Rochester, NY, USA.

As a result, camera systems with high sensitivity and/or image-averaging capabilities (with alignment to account for eye movements) [24] are required to record the FAF with acceptable signal/noise ratios using safe retinal exposure levels. Confocal scanning laser ophthalmoscopy (cSLO) [25] optimally addressed these requirements and was used by Fred Fitzke (London) in the first clinical FAF imaging system [26, 27]. Subsequent developments using different scanning laser ophthalmoscope (SLO) systems [28, 29] further opened the field of FAF imaging (Fig. 2.1a). Continuous technical innovations have resulted in higher quality images [30], and the recent introduction of two-photon fluorescence imaging [31] and adaptive optics technology [32] has led to high magnification imaging in which individual RPE cells can be resolved because of the autofluorescence of LF (Fig. 2.1b).

The excitation wavelength used in FAF imaging is generally, but not always [32–35], 488 nm (argon laser). Compared with longer excitation wavelengths, this is probably not the best wavelength for FAF imaging because the ocular media and the macular pigment substantially absorb light at that wavelength. Absorption by macular pigment prevents clear visualization of the foveal RPE. Furthermore, short wavelengths are more susceptible to photochemical damage to the retina [36].

2.4
Influence of Crystalline Lens Absorption

Measurements of autofluorescence from the fundus are affected by absorption in the lens and other ocular media. For example, an excitation at 488 nm would be attenuated, on average, by a factor of 1.4 and 2.7 for ages 20 and 70 years, respectively [37]. The autofluorescence emission is also attenuated but to a lesser extent because it occurs at longer wavelengths (factors 1.05 and 1.14, respectively, when averaged over the emission from 500 to 800 nm). Thus, correction methods need to be used to account for this light loss if absolute FAF levels are needed. This light loss can be estimated for each subject by psychophysical [38] or reflectometric [39, 40] methods. Alternatively, algorithms predicting the average light loss at a given age can be used in population studies [37, 41].

2.5
Spatial Distribution of FAF

FAF images from subjects with normal retinal status (Fig. 2.1a) show a central dark area caused by the combined attenuation of the autofluorescence by RPE melanin (this tends to be located on the apical side of the RPE cells [42]) and by macular pigment (which absorbs strongly for wavelengths shorter than 520 nm [43]). The retinal vessels are dark and often show a parallel narrow band of higher autofluorescence that may be caused by refraction effects at the vessel walls. The autofluorescence seen in macular holes has intensity similar to that in the surrounding field; the autofluorescence is affected by absorption of visual pigments [44], and its emission spectrum does not show any blood signature from choriocapillaris. These observations are consistent with RPE LF being the principal source of FAF [23].

Lipofuscin and its autofluorescence are low at the fovea, increase gradually to a maximum at 7–13° from the fovea, and then decrease toward the periphery [45, 46]. FAF is not symmetrically distributed around the fovea (Fig. 2.2): The signal is maximal at about 12° temporally and superiorly and lower inferiorly and nasally, where it is maximal at about 7–8° from the fovea. The FAF distribution roughly matches the distribution of rod photoreceptors [47], which is not surprising since LF derives from precursors within phagocytosed photoreceptor outer segments. What is surprising, however, is that the distribution does not reflect the narrow distribution of cones at the fovea. Instead, FAF imaging at 550 nm reveals a shallow minimum in autofluorescence with no systematic increase in the signal corresponding to the narrow cone distribution [34]. The rate of LF formation from cones may be slower, as suggested by the observation in Rhesus monkeys that the number of foveal cone-derived phagosomes in the RPE was only one-third of the number of extrafoveal rod-derived phagosomes [48]. Other effects such as high absorption by RPE melanin at the fovea, cone/rod differences in the fractional content of indigestible materials in the phagosomes, and spatially dependent protection by the macular pigment could also play a role in reducing foveal LF formation.

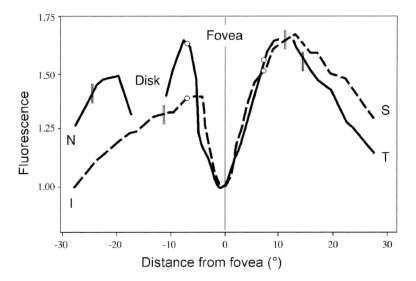

Fig. 2.2 Spatial distribution of fundus autofluorescence (FAF) based on measurements along the horizontal (nasal-temporal) and vertical (superior-inferior) meridians (data from about 40 subjects) [46]. The FAF is expressed relative to that at the fovea. The *double lines* on each meridian indicate the intersection of the rod ring (high rod density) with the meridians [47]. The FAF distribution roughly corresponds with the location of that rod ring, except for the inferior meridian

2.6

Spectral Properties of FAF

FAF can be excited between 430 and 600 nm, but its highest efficiency is obtained with excitation wavelengths from 480 to 510 nm. The emission spectrum is broad (480–800 nm) and maximal in the 600–640 nm region of the spectrum, shifting slightly toward the deep red with increasing excitation wavelength. Compared with the spectra measured 7° temporal to the fovea, the foveal spectra are attenuated, even outside the absorption range of macular pigment (Fig. 2.3). This is due in part to the lower amount of LF in the foveal area, the attenuation by RPE melanin that is denser in the fovea than in the parafoveal area [45], and the absorption of the excitation light by macular pigment (for wavelengths shorter than 550 nm). The foveal-parafoveal differences in the shape of the excitation spectra are the basis of the two-wavelength FAF method to measure macular pigment (see chapter 6.4)[49].

Comparison of the emission spectra of A2E [7] and those of FAF show roughly similarly shaped spectra with maxima at 600 nm and 620 nm, respectively (excitation wavelength: 400–430 nm). However, the excitation spectrum of A2E is much narrower and shifted toward shorter wavelengths compared with those from the fundus (after correction for media absorption) [50]. This implies that A2E is only one of the LF fluorophores responsible for FAF. Other secondary LF fluorophores (iso-A2E,

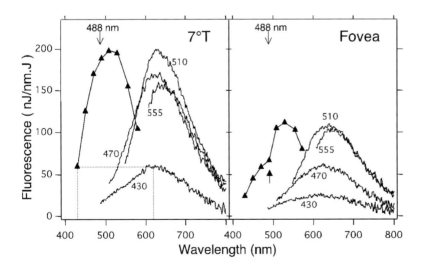

Fig. 2.3 Fluorescence spectra measured in a 52-year-old normal subject at 7° temporal to the fovea and at the fovea (sampling: 2° diameter). *Continuous lines* indicate emission spectra (excitation wavelength as indicated), and *lines with filled triangles* indicate excitation spectrum for emission at 620 nm. The excitation spectrum is not measured but is constructed from the fluorescence at 620 nm and plotted against the excitation wavelength. The foveal spectra are lower than at 7° temporal, particularly for excitation wavelengths shorter than 490 nm (*arrow*) where absorption of the excitation light by macular pigment is revealed

ATR dimer conjugate [51]) cannot account for the observed differences. It is likely that unidentified LF fluorophores that are not soluble in solvents normally used to extract LF contribute to the autofluorescence detected in vivo.

Evidence of secondary non-LF fluorophores comes from changes in the shape of the emission spectra observed with retinal location (Fig. 2.3) and with age (Fig. 2.4). There is an age-related blue shift and distortion of the emission spectra, characterized by a relative increase of FAF in the 500–540 nm spectral region (Fig. 2.4). This shift is most pronounced in AMD patients and when measurements are made on distinct drusen or in areas with numerous drusen [52]. The spectral shift at older ages is probably due to the autofluorescence of drusen and/or Bruch's membrane deposits (BMD). Computations using model spectral templates predict that the BMD autofluorescence could be as high as 30% of the LF autofluorescence in the 500–540-nm emission range for an excitation at 510 nm [53]. For an excitation at 488 nm, which is usually used in FAF imaging, BMD fluorescence could contribute 22±22% of the total FAF detected between 500 and 700 nm. This could, in part, explain the varying appearance of drusen in FAF images in AMD patients.

The spectral distortion observed for the young fovea (Fig. 2.4) is also characterized by a relative increase in the 500–540 nm emission range. The autofluorescence from LF

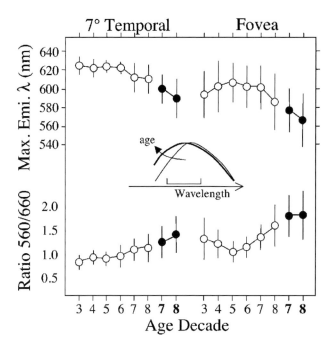

Fig. 2.4 Age-related changes in the shape of the emission spectrum (excitation: 470 nm), characterized by its peak wavelength (*top*) and the ratio of the fundus autofluorescence at 560 nm and that at 660 nm (*bottom*). The spectra were corrected to account for absorption of the ocular media. A sketch in the middle of the plot illustrates the effect. *Open circles* represent normal subjects, and *filled circles* represent age-related macular degeneration patients

is very low at young ages, and any secondary fluorophore may therefore become significant. This fluorescence is believed to originate anterior to the macular pigment and could emanate from the vitreous, the lens, and/or the macular pigment itself [54].

2.7
Age Relationship of FAF

In-vivo FAF increases significantly with age [20, 23, 27, 46], consistent with observations from ex-vivo studies [55, 56]. The rate and time course of this increase vary among different studies, probably as a result of differences in population selection, technique, correction method for media absorption, and other factors [46]. The increase of FAF with age for a population of normal subjects (Fig. 2.5) shows a large but constant variability (the coefficient of variation per decade of age is about 25 and 28%). The foveal autofluorescence increases similarly with age. Indeed, the ratio of the autofluorescence at the fovea to that at 7° temporal to the fovea does not vary with age.

The decrease in FAF observed above age 70 has not been demonstrated in other studies although only a few showed significant increases at old age. The decrease in fluorescence at ages greater than 70 years could result, in part, from an undercorrection by our lens optical density estimates, from the presence of incipient atrophy, or from changes in fluorescence efficiency [57]. Indeed, over 40% of the fluorescent granules in that age group are melanolipofuscin granules [1], and these have been shown to be less fluorescent than LF granules [58].

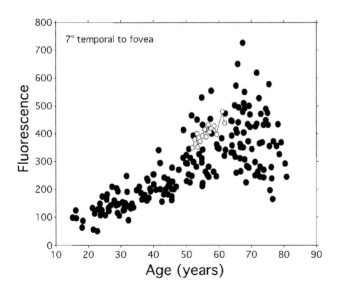

Fig. 2.5 Age-related change in fundus autofluorescence for subjects with normal retinal status. The excitation wavelength was 550 nm, and the fluorescence was measured in the 610–630 nm spectral range. The data were corrected to account for absorption by the ocular media. The *open circles* represent longitudinal measurements in one subject over a period of about 10 years

2.8
Near-Infrared FAF

In addition to the FAF images recorded with short-wavelength excitation (SW-FAF) images, autofluorescence images with near-infrared (NIR) excitation can also be obtained (NIR-FAF images) [59, 60]. The confocal SLO (Heidelberg Retina Angiograph, HRA; Heidelberg Engineering, Heidelberg, Germany) is operated in the indocyanine green (ICG) mode (excitation: 790 nm; detection above 800 nm) to produce a weak signal that is 60–100 times less intense than that obtained with SW-FAF imaging. The large dynamic range of the SLO, however, allows imaging, albeit with low contrast, that appears to provide different information than SW-FAF images.

The most striking feature of NIR-FAF images of a normal retina is an area of high autofluorescence that is roughly centered on the fovea (Fig. 2.6a) and corresponds to the central area of higher RPE melanin seen in color images [60]. Higher NIR-FAF

SW-AF   NIR-AF

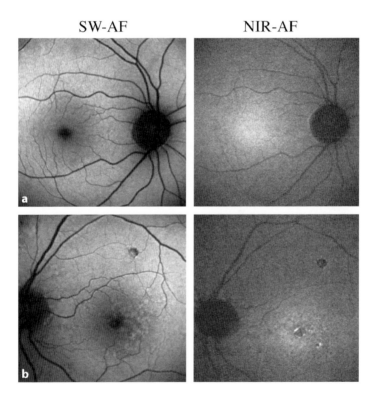

Fig. 2.6 Autofluorescence images obtained with a confocal scanning laser ophthalmoscope (HRAc, Heidelberg Engineering) using 488 nm short-wavelength and 787 nm near-infrared as excitation wavelengths. **a** Images from a 44-year-old subject with normal retinal status. **b** Images from an 81-year-old age-related macular degeneration patient with drusen and early atrophic changes in the fovea. Hyperpigmentation exhibits high autofluorescence in both imaging modes

also emanates from choroidal pigment (nevi, outer layers), from the pigment epithelium and stroma of the iris, and from hyperpigmentation (Fig. 2.6b). The latter are clumps of stacked or hyperpigmented (LF, melanin, and melanolipofuscin) RPE cells in the subretinal and sub-RPE space [61]. Similar to SW-FAF, low NIR-FAF is observed in geographic atrophy, indicating that the autofluorescence originates in part from the RPE.

These observations suggest that NIR-FAF originates from melanin and/or from compounds closely related to melanin (oxidized melanin, melanolipofuscin) [60]. Small contributions from other fluorophores, including LF fluorophores, cannot be excluded at this point.

Because choroidal melanin contributes to the NIR-FAF, one can expect the contrast of retinal fluorescent highlights to be higher when the choroidal background is low or when there is little melanin in the choroidal layers (light irides). Indeed, the contrast of the central bright area is higher in subjects with light irides than in those with dark irides [60].

2.9
Conclusions

Fundus autofluorescence derives principally from RPE LF as evidenced by its spatial distribution, its spectral characteristics, and its relationship with age. Additional autofluorescence may originate from BMD and drusen, but this has not yet been sufficiently characterized to provide specific information about the type or content of drusen. Near-infrared autofluorescence appears to emanate from melanin or from compounds closely related to melanin. Additional spectral studies, as well as long-time follow-up in pathological conditions, will be important for a better understanding of the unresolved biophysical issues and particularly of the biological changes associated with aging and pathology.

References

1.   Feeney-Burns, L, Hilderbrand, ES, Eldridge, S (1984) Aging human RPE: Morphometric analysis of macular, equatorial, and peripheral cells. Invest Ophthalmol Vis Sci 25:195–200

2.   Boulton, M, Dontsov, A, Jarvis-Evans, J et al. (1993) Lipofuscin is a photoinducible free radical generator. J Photochem Photobiol B 19:201–204

3.   Holz, FG, Schutt, F, Kopitz, J et al. (1999) Inhibition of lysosomal degradative functions in RPE cells by a retinoid component of lipofuscin. Invest Ophthalmol Vis Sci 40:737–743

4.   Schutt, F, Davies, S, Kopitz, J et al. (2000) Photodamage to human RPE cells by A2-E, a retinoid component of lipofuscin. Invest Ophthalmol Vis Sci 41:2303–2308

5.   Sparrow, JR, Cai, B, Fishkin, N et al. (2003) A2E, a fluorophore of RPE lipofuscin: can it cause RPE degeneration? Adv Exp Med Biol 533:205–211

6.   Sparrow, JR, Fishkin, N, Zhou, J et al. (2003) A2E, a byproduct of the visual cycle. Vision Res 43:2983–2990

7.   Sparrow, JR, Nakanishi, K, Parish, CA (2000) The lipofuscin fluorophore A2E mediates blue light-induced damage to retinal pigmented epithelial cells. Invest Ophthalmol Vis Sci 41:1981–1989

8.   Sparrow, JR, Zhou, J, Ben-Shabat, S et al. (2002) Involvement of oxidative mechanisms in blue-light-induced damage to A2E-laden RPE. Invest Ophthalmol Vis Sci 43:1222–1227

9.   Sparrow, JR, Zhou, J, Cai, B (2003) DNA is a target of the photodynamic effects elicited in A2E-laden RPE by blue-light illumination. Invest Ophthalmol Vis Sci 44:2245–2251

10. Eagle, RC, Lucier, AC, Bernadino, VB et al. (1980) Retinal pigment epithelial abnormalities in fundus flavimaculatus: a light and electron microscopic study. Ophthalmology 87:1189–1200

11. Delori, FC, Staurenghi, G, Arend, O et al. (1995) In-vivo measurement of lipofuscin in Stargardt's disease/fundus flavimaculatus. Invest Ophthalmol Vis Sci 36:2331–2337

12. von Rückmann, A, Fitzke, FW, Bird, AC (1997) In vivo fundus autofluorescence in macular dystrophies. Arch Ophthalmol 115:609–615

13. Allikmets, R, Singh, N, Sun, H et al. (1997) A photoreceptor cell-specific ATP-binding transporter gene (*ABCR*) is mutated in recessive Stargardt macular dystrophy. Nature Genetics 15:236–245

14. Azarian, SM, Travis, GH (1997) The photoreceptor rim protein is an ABC transporter encoded by the gene for recessive Stargardt's disease (ABCR). FEBS Lett 409:247–252

15. Weng, J, Mata, NL, Azarian, SM et al. (1999) Insights into the function of Rim protein in photoreceptors and etiology of Stargardt's disease from the phenotype in abcr knockout mice. Cell 98:13–23

16. Kim, SR, Fishkin, N, Kong, J et al. (2004) Rpe65 Leu450Met variant is associated with reduced levels of the retinal pigment epithelium lipofuscin fluorophores A2E and iso-A2E. Proc Natl Acad Sci USA 101:11668–11672

17. Kramer, F, White, K, Pauleikhoff, D et al. (2000) Mutations in the VMD2 gene are associated with juvenile-onset vitelliform macular dystrophy (Best disease) and adult vitelliform macular dystrophy but not age-related macular degeneration. Eur J Hum Genet 8:286–292

18. Graydon, RJ, Jolly, RD (1984) Ceroid lipofuscinosis (Batten's disease). Invest Ophthal 25:294–301

19. Delori, FC, Bursell, S-E, Yoshida, A et al. (1985) Vitreous fluorophotometry in diabetics: study of artifactual contributions. Graefe's Arch Clin Exp Ophthalmol 222:215–218

20. Kitagawa, K, Nishida, S, Ogura, Y (1989) In vivo quantification of autofluorescence in human retinal pigment epithelium. Ophthalmologica 199:116–121

21. Delori, FC (1992) Fluorophotometer for noninvasive measurement of RPE lipofuscin. Noninvasive assessment of the visual system. OSA Technical Digest 1:164–167

22. Delori, FC (1994) Spectrophotometer for noninvasive measurement of intrinsic fluorescence and reflectance of the ocular fundus. Applied Optics 33:7439–7452

23. Delori, FC, Dorey, CK, Staurenghi, G et al. (1995) In vivo fluorescence of the ocular fundus exhibits retinal pigment epithelium lipofuscin characteristics. Invest Ophthalmol Vis Sci 36:718–729

24. Wade, AR, Fitzke, FW (1998) A fast, robust pattern recognition system for low light level image registration and its application to retinal imaging. Optics Express 3:190–197

25. Webb, RH, Hughes, GW, Delori, FC (1987) Confocal scanning laser ophthalmoscope. Appl Opt 26:1492–1449

26. von Rückmann, A, Fitzke, FW, Bird, AC (1995) Distribution of fundus autofluorescence with a scanning laser ophthalmoscope. Br J Ophthalmol 119:543–562

27. von Rückmann, A, Fitzke, FW, Bird, AC (1997) Fundus Autofluorescence in age-related macular disease imaged with a laser scanning ophthalmoscope. Invest Ophthalmol Vis Sci 38:478–486

28. Solbach, U, Keilhauer, C, Knabben, H et al. (1997) Imaging of retinal autofluorescence in patients with age-related macular degeneration. Retina 17:385–389

29. Holz, FG, Bellmann, C, Margaritidis, M et al. (1999) Patterns of increased in vivo fundus autofluorescence in the junctional zone of geographic atrophy of the retinal pigment epithelium associated with age-related macular degeneration. Graefes Arch Clin Exp Ophthalmol 237:145–152

30. Bindewald, A, Jorzik, JJ, Loesch, A et al. (2004) Visualization of retinal pigment epithelial cells in vivo using digital high-resolution confocal scanning laser ophthalmoscopy. Am J Ophthalmol 137:556–558

31. Bindewald-Wittich, A, Han, M, Schmitz-Valckenberg, S et al. (2006) Two-photon-excited fluorescence imaging of human RPE cells with a femtosecond Ti:sapphire laser. Invest Ophthalmol Vis Sci 47:4553–4557

32. Gray, DC, Merigan, W, Wolfing, JI et al. (2006) In vivo fluorescence imaging of primate retinal ganglion cells and retinal pigment epithelial cells. Optics Express 14:7144–7158

33. Delori, FC, Fleckner, MR, Goger, DG et al. (2000) Autofluorescence distribution associated with drusen in age-related macular degeneration. Invest Ophthalmol Vis Sci 41:496–504

34. Delori, FC, Goger, DG, Keilhauer, CN et al. (2006) Bimodal spatial distribution of macular pigment: evidence of a gender relationship. J Opt Soc Am A Opt Image Sci Vis 23:521–538

35. Spaide, RF (2003) Fundus autofluorescence and age-related macular degeneration. Ophthalmology 110:392–399

36. ANSI, American National Standard for Safe Use of Lasers (ANSI 136.1) (2000). In: ANSI 136.1-2000. The Laser Institute of America, Orlando, FL, USA

37. Pokorny, J, Smith, VC, Lutze, M (1987) Aging of the human lens. Appl Opt 26:1437–1440

38. Savage, GL, Johnson, CA, Howard, DL (2001) A comparison of noninvasive objective and subjective measurements of the optical density of human ocular media. Optom Vis Sci 78:386–395

39. Delori, FC, Burns, SA (1996) Fundus reflectance and the measurement of crystalline lens density. J Opt Soc Am A 13:215–226

40. Berendschot, TT, Broekmans, WM, Klopping-Ketelaars, IA et al. (2002) Lens aging in relation to nutritional determinants and possible risk factors for age-related cataract. Arch Ophthalmol 120:1732–1737

41. van de Kraats, J, van Norren, D (2007) Optical density of the young and aging human ocular media in the visible and the UV. J Opt Soc Am A Ophthalmol Image Sci Vis (in press)

42. Feeney-Burns, L, Berman, ER, Rothman, H (1980) Lipofuscin of human retinal pigment epithelium. Am J Ophthalmol 90:783–791

43. Bone, RA, Landrum, JT, Cains, A (1992) Optical density spectra of the macular pigment in vivo and in vitro. Vision Res 32:105–110

44. Prieto, PM, McLellan, JS, Burns, SA (2005) Investigating the light absorption in a single pass through the photoreceptor layer by means of the lipofuscin fluorescence. Vision Res 45:1957–1965

45. Weiter, JJ, Delori, FC, Wing, G et al. (1986) Retinal pigment epithelial lipofuscin and melanin and choroidal melanin in human eyes. Invest Ophthalmol Vis Sci 27:145–152

46. Delori, FC, Goger, DG, Dorey, CK (2001) Age-related accumulation and spatial distribution of lipofuscin in RPE of normal subjects. Invest Ophthalmol Vis Sci 42:1855–1866

47. Curcio, CA, Sloan, KR, Kalina, RE et al. (1990) Human photoreceptor topography. J Comp Neural 292:497–523

48. Anderson, DH, Fisher, SK, Erickson, PA et al. (1980) Rod and cone disc shedding in the rhesus monkey retina: a quantitative study. Exp Eye Res 30:559–574

49. Delori, FC, Goger, DG, Hammond, BR et al. (2001) Macular pigment density measured by autofluorescence spectrometry: comparison with reflectometry and heterochromatic flicker photometry. J Opt Soc Am A Opt Image Sci Vis 18:1212–1230

50. Delori, FC, Goger, DG, Sparrow, JR (2003) Spectral characteristics of lipofuscin autofluorescence in RPE cells of donor eyes. Invest Ophthalmol Vis Sci 44:1715

51. Fishkin, NE, Sparrow, JR, Allikmets, R et al. (2005) Isolation and characterization of a retinal pigment epithelial cell fluorophore: an all-trans-retinal dimer conjugate. Proc Natl Acad Sci USA 102:7091–7096

52. Arend, OA, Weiter, JJ, Goger, DG et al. (1995) In-vivo fundus-fluoreszenz-messungen bei patienten mit alterabhangiger makulardegeneration. Ophthalmologie 92:647–653

53. Delori, FC, RPE lipofuscin in aging and age related macular degeneration. In: Piccolino, FC and Coscas, G (1998) Retinal pigment epithelium and macular diseases. Kluwer Academic Publishers, Dordrecht, The Netherlands

54. Gellermann, W, Ermakov, IV, Ermakova, MR et al. (2002) In vivo resonant Raman measurement of macular carotenoid pigments in the young and the aging human retina. J Opt Soc Am A Opt Image Sci Vis 19:1172–1186

55. Wing, GL, Blanchard, GC, Weiter, JJ (1978) The topography and age relationship of lipofuscin concentration in the retinal pigment epithelium. Invest Ophthalmol Vis Sci 17:601–607

56. Okubo, A, Rosa, RH, Jr., Bunce, CV et al. (1999) The relationships of age changes in retinal pigment epithelium and Bruch's membrane. Invest Ophthalmol Vis Sci 40:443–449

57. Boulton, MD, Dayhaw-Barker, F, Ramponi, P, Cubeddu, R (1990) Age-related changes in the morphology, absorption and fluorescence of melanosomes and lipofuscin granules of the retinal pigment epithelium. Vision Res 30:1291–1303

58. Docchio, F, Boulton, M, Cubeddu, R et al. (1991) Age-related changes in the fluorescence of melanin and lipofuscin granules of the retinal pigment epithelium: a time-resolved fluorescence spectroscopy study. J Photochem Photobiol 54:247–253

59. Weinberger, AWA, Lappas, A, Kirschkamp, T et al. (2006) Fundus near-infrared fluorescence is correlated to fundus near-infrared reflectance. Invest Ophthal Vis Sci 42:3098–3108

60. Keilhauer, CN, Delori, FC (2006) Near-infrared autofluorescence imaging of the fundus: visualization of ocular melanin. Invest Ophthalmol Vis Sci 47:3556–3564

61. Sarks, JP, Sarks, SH, Killingsworth, MC (1988) Evolution of geographic atrophy of the retinal pigment epithelium. Eye 2:552–577

Fundus Autofluorescence Imaging with the Confocal Scanning Laser Ophthalmoscope

3

Steffen Schmitz-Valckenberg, Fred W. Fitzke, Frank G. Holz

3.1
The Confocal Scanning Laser Ophthalmoscope (cSLO)

The confocal scanning laser ophthalmoscope (cSLO), which was originally developed by Webb and coworkers, projects a low-power laser beam on the retina (Fig. 3.1) [11]. The laser beam is deflected by oscillating mirrors to sequentially scan the fundus in x and y directions. The intensity of the reflected light at each point, after passing through the confocal pinhole, is registered by means of a detector, and a two-dimensional image is subsequently generated. Confocal optics ensures that out-of-focus light (i.e., light originating outside the adjusted focal plane but within the light beam) is suppressed; thus, the image contrast is enhanced. This suppression increases with the distance from the focal plane, and signals from sources anterior to the retina (i.e., the lens or the cornea) are effectively reduced. In addition to focusing of the structure of interest, the optics also allows correction for refractive errors.

3.2
FAF Imaging with the cSLO

Fundus autofluorescence imaging (FAF) with the cSLO was initially described by von Rückmann and coworkers in 1995 (see Chap. 4, Fig. 4.1) [10]. Using a cSLO, they were able to visualize the topographic distribution of retinal pigment epithelium (RPE) lipofuscin over large retinal areas in vivo.

In comparison to fundus reflectance or fluorescence angiography, the FAF signal is characterized by a very low intensity. To reduce background noise and to enhance image contrast, a series of several single FAF images is usually recorded [2, 5, 8–10]. Subsequently, the mean image (usually out of 4–16 frames) is calculated, and pixel values are normalized. Because of a high rate of up to 16 frames per second and the high sensitivity of the cSLO, FAF imaging can be recorded in a non-time-consuming manner and at low excitation energies that are well below the maximum laser retinal irradiance limits established by the American National Standards Institute and other international standards (ANSI Z136.1; 1993) [1].

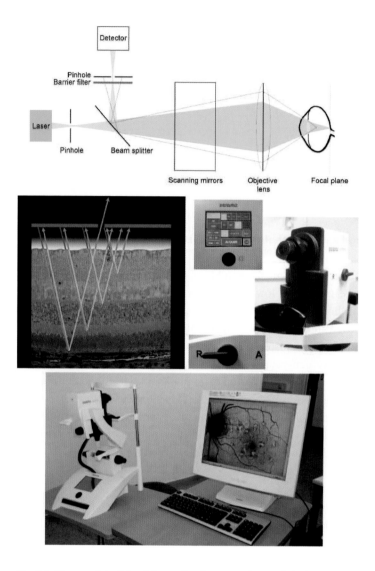

Fig. 3.1 *Top row:* Principle of the confocal scanning laser ophthalmoscope. The laser is focused through a pinhole diaphragm to the focal plane (*blue light*). The reflected laser light is separated by a beam splitter from the incident laser beam path and is deflected through a second pinhole to reach a photosensitive detector (*yellow light*). Light originating outside the focal plane (*red light*) is effectively suppressed by the pinhole. *Middle row left:* Schematic illustration of the confocal optics. Light originating from the precise plane of focus (here, the retinal pigment epithelium) can pass through the pinhole and reach the detector. In contrast, light originating in the light beam but out of the focal plane is blocked. *Middle row right:* The Heidelberg Retina Angiograph (HRA 2) with laser scanning camera, imaged from the patient side. The image acquisition procedures are controlled by a touch panel, and the filter wheel easily permits a change from reflectance (*R*) to autofluorescence (*A*) mode by placing the barrier filter in front of the detector. *Lower row:* The Heidelberg Retina Angiograph (HRA 2) in the clinical setting imaged from the operator's side. During the acquisition, images are immediately digitized and displayed on a computer screen. This allows adjustment of settings and optimization of the image in real time

Three different cSLO systems have so far been used for obtaining FAF images: Heidelberg Retina Angiograph [HRA classic, HRA 2 (Fig. 3.1) and Spectralis HRA, Heidelberg Engineering, Heidelberg, Germany (Fig. 3.2)]; Rodenstock cSLO (RcSLO; Rodenstock, Weco, Düsseldorf, Germany), and Zeiss prototype SM 30 4024 (ZcSLO; Zeiss, Oberkochen, Germany). The latter two are not commercially available. For FAF imaging, these instruments use an excitation wavelength of 488 nm generated by an argon or solid-state laser. In order to block the reflected light and to allow the autofluorescence light to pass, a wide band-pass barrier filter with a short wavelength cutoff is inserted in front of the detector. The cut-off edge of the barrier filter is at 500 nm for the HRA classic and HRA 2, 515 nm for the RcSLO, and 521 nm for the ZcSLO. Despite clinically useful FAF imaging with all three systems, Bellmann and coworkers have reported significant differences in image contrast and brightness as well as in the range of gray values as important indicators for image quality between these three cSLOs [3]. These differences are important when comparing FAF findings from different imaging devices.

Modern cSLO systems achieve high-contrast images of various structures of the posterior segment [8]. With a current commercially available cSLO system and in the presence of clear optical media, good patient cooperation, and sufficient lipofuscin granule density, the in-vivo visualization of the polygonal RPE cell pattern in the outer macula area has been demonstrated [6]. The lateral resolution of the cSLO is limited by the numerical aperture of the optical system, which is given by the beam diameter at the pupil (typically 3 mm) and the focal length of the eye. In principle, the numerical aperture could be increased by dilating the pupil and expanding the laser beam. However, in practice this does not result in improvement as the optical quality of the eye decreases for larger pupil diameters because of high-order aberrations. Therefore, increasing the digital pixel resolution (number of pixels per area) with current available systems will not improve the resolution of the actual fundus image, but rather will result in an artificial, high-resolution, posterized image. To improve visualization of fine retinal structures, promising approaches include the use of adaptive optics to better correct for the optical properties of the eye and the application of two-photon excited fluorescence to reduce the signal-to-noise ratio and enlarge the sensing depth [4, 7].

The technical details of the only commercially available cSLO for FAF imaging at the time of publication, the Heidelberg Retina Angiograph 2, are summarized in Table 3.1.

Table 3.1 Technical details for fundus autofluorescence (FAF) imaging with the Heidelberg Retina Angiograph 2, a confocal scanning laser ophthalmoscopy system

Reflectance imaging	$\lambda = 488$ nm (blue light) $\lambda = 830$ nm (near-infrared)
Autofluorescence imaging (blue light)	Excitation: $\lambda = 488$ nm, emission $\lambda > 500$ nm

Table 3.1 *(Continued)* Technical details for fundus autofluorescence (FAF) imaging with the Heidelberg Retina Angiograph 2, a confocal scanning laser ophthalmoscopy system

Near-infrared autofluorescence imaging ("ICG mode")	Excitation: λ = 790 nm, emission λ > 800 nm
Image size (in pixels at 15°, 20°, and 30°)	768×768, 1,024×1,024, 1,536×1,536 (high-resolution mode) 384×384, 512×512, 768×768 (high-speed mode)
Digital pixel resolution	10 μm/pixel (high-speed mode) 5 μm/pixel (high-resolution mode)
Optical resolution	Maximum 5 μm–10 μm, depending on optical quality of the patient's eye
Frame size (in degrees)	30×30 (standard) (between 15×15 and 55×55)
Focus range (in dpt)	−24 to +40
Frame rate per second	Up to 16
Additional features for FAF imaging	Composite mode Automatic real-time image averaging

3.3
Combination of cSLO Imaging with Spectral-Domain Optical Coherence Tomography

A further development of the cSLO (Spectralis HRA + OCT, Heidelberg Engineering, Heidelberg, Germany) includes combination with spectral-domain optical coherence tomography (OCT) in one instrument. This new imaging device allows for simultaneous cSLO and OCT recordings. A major advantage is that any lateral eye movement can be detected in real time with the cSLO system and fed into the scanning system of the OCT modality. This allows a very precise registration of the OCT A-scans. In addition, with the use of any cSLO imaging mode (reflectance, FAF, or angiography) as the reference image, retinal locations seen on the fundus image can be mapped to cross-sectional OCT findings. Volumetric assessment of retinal structures can also be achieved. Three different clinical examples are illustrated in Fig. 3.2. Because of the high resolution of Spectralis OCT technology, "optical biopsies" of the retina can be obtained with visualization of different retinal layers and localized pathologies.

Alterations in FAF intensities, such as areas with increased intensity, can be compared with the spatial distribution of RPE changes such as drusen (Fig. 3.2b).

This imaging device may give further insights and clues into the pathogenesis and understanding of macular and retinal diseases. It may also be helpful for observing patients over time and for monitoring therapeutic interventions.

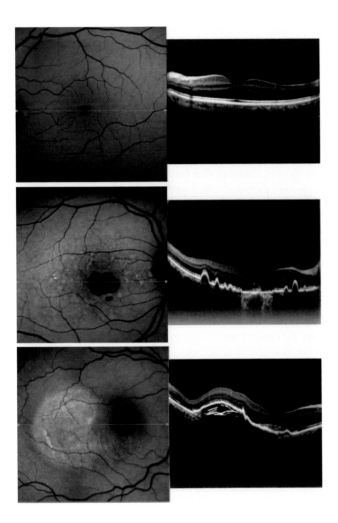

Fig. 3.2 Three examples of simultaneous fundus autofluorescence (FAF) imaging and optical coherence tomography (OCT) imaging with the combined confocal scanning laser ophthalmoscope and spectral-domain, high-resolution OCT (Spectralis HRA/OCT, Heidelberg Engineering). The *green line* indicates the position of the OCT cross-section. *Top row:* FAF and OCT images in a normal eye. *Middle row:* Geographic atrophy secondary to age-related macular degeneration. *Bottom row:* Pigment epithelial detachment in the presence of an occult choroidal neovascularization

References

1. American National Standards Institute (2000) American national standard for the safe use of lasers: ANSI Z136.1. Laser Institute of America, Orlando, FL

2. Bellmann, C, Holz, FG, Schapp, O, et al. (1997) [Topography of fundus autofluorescence with a new confocal scanning laser ophthalmoscope]. Ophthalmologe 94:385–391

3. Bellmann, C, Rubin, GS, Kabanarou, SA, et al. (2003) Fundus autofluorescence imaging compared with different confocal scanning laser ophthalmoscopes. Br J Ophthalmol 87:1381–1386

4. Bindewald-Wittich, A, Han, M, Schmitz-Valckenberg, S, et al. (2006) Two-photon-excited fluorescence imaging of human RPE cells with a femtosecond Ti:sapphire laser. Invest Ophthalmol Vis Sci 47:4553–4557

5. Bindewald, A, Jorzik, JJ, Roth, F, Holz, FG (2005) [cSLO digital fundus autofluorescence imaging]. Ophthalmologe 102:259–264

6. Bindewald, A, Jorzik, JJ, Loesch, A, et al. (2004) Visualization of retinal pigment epithelial cells in vivo using digital high-resolution confocal scanning laser ophthalmoscopy. Am J Ophthalmol 137:556–558

7. Gray, DC, Merigan, W, Wolfing, JI, et al. (2006) In vivo fluorescence imaging of primate retinal ganglion cells and retinal pigment epithelial cells. Opt Express 14:7144–7158

8. Jorzik, JJ, Bindewald, A, Dithmar, S, Holz, FG (2005) Digital simultaneous fluorescein and indocyanine green angiography, autofluorescence, and red-free imaging with a solid-state laser-based confocal scanning laser ophthalmoscope. Retina 25:405–416

9. Solbach, U, Keilhauer, C, Knabben, H, Wolf, S (1997) Imaging of retinal autofluorescence in patients with age-related macular degeneration. Retina 17:385–389

10. von Rückmann, A, Fitzke, FW, Bird, AC (1995) Distribution of fundus autofluorescence with a scanning laser ophthalmoscope. Br J Ophthalmol 79:407–412

11. Webb, RH, Hughes, GW, Delori, FC (1987) Confocal scanning laser ophthalmoscope. Appl Optics 26:1492–1499

How To Obtain the Optimal Fundus Autofluorescence Image with the Confocal Scanning Laser Ophthalmoscope

4

Steffen Schmitz-Valckenberg, Vy Luong, Fred W. Fitzke, Frank G. Holz

4.1
Basic Considerations

The aim of this chapter is to give a brief overview of obtaining fundus autofluorescence (FAF) images with the confocal scanning laser ophthalmoscope (cSLO) and to illustrate some common pitfalls that can occur during image acquisition.

As with any imaging method, the quality of FAF images is of utmost importance in order to gain optimal information from these recordings. Poor image quality may give rise to misinterpretation or may even render FAF image interpretation impossible. The use of a standardized protocol and the consideration of some basic principles can significantly improve image quality and facilitate analysis of FAF images [2, 3].

The cSLO scans the retina continuously; the actual image is immediately digitized and visualized on a computer screen. Settings such as orientation and position of the laser scanning camera, laser intensity, detector sensitivity, and refractive correction can be easily adjusted during the acquisition process and in real time by the operator. This way of image recording differs greatly from image acquisition with the usual fundus camera. It should be also noted that the high sensitivity and relatively low light levels (intensity per retinal area) of the cSLO make it possible to continuously scan the retina and to visualize the fundus image in real time without exposing the patient's retina to the high light levels required by an equivalent fundus camera system.

4.2
Reflectance Before Autofluorescence Imaging

Although light intensities of the cSLO are well below the established safety levels, the exposure time to the patient's retina should be kept to a minimum [1]. The examiner should also take into account that blue light—even at these low intensity levels—is much more uncomfortable for the examined patient than near-infrared light. Therefore, the orientation of the camera position and a first focusing should be initially performed in the near-infrared reflectance mode (Fig. 4.1a). Subsequently, the examiner should switch to the blue-light laser. Different chromatic aberrations between near-infrared and blue light can cause a small focus difference. To obtain best-quality FAF images, the focus of the optics should therefore be slightly readjusted in the blue light (or so-called red-free) reflectance mode in order to compensate for the wavelength-dependent refractive power of the optics and the eye (Fig. 4.1b). Finally, the barrier filter can be put in front of the detector, and FAF images be acquired (Fig. 4.1c).

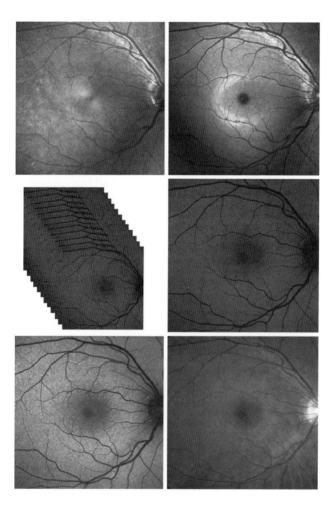

Fig. 4. 1 Illustration of different cSLO images obtained through the acquisition process and comparison with a normal fundus photograph for a normal right eye. **a** *(top left)* Near-infrared reflectance image. **b** *(top right)* Blue-light (or so-called red-free) reflectance image. **c** *(middle left)* Selection of 12 single fundus autofluorescence (FAF) images of good quality. **d** *(middle right)* Mean image obtained from the 12 single images. **e** *(bottom left)* Final FAF image following normalizing of pixel values of the previous figure. **f** *(bottom right)* Fundus photograph of the same eye obtained with the fundus camera

4.3

Image Alignment and Calculation of Mean Image

As discussed in Chap. 3, the autofluorescence signal has a very low intensity and is therefore characterized by a relatively low signal-to-noise ratio. This ratio can be improved by averaging a series of images. Theoretically, the signal-to-noise ratio increases by a factor of $\sqrt{n}$, where n is the number of images to be averaged. For example, the averaging of a series of nine images will improve the signal-to-noise ratio by a factor of three. Typically, a series of 8–16 images is averaged (Fig. 4.1c). Using more images is usually not practical in the clinical setting for various reasons. First, due to mere mathematical reasons, the number of images required to enhance the signal-to-noise ratio by a certain factor increases by the square of this number. For example, to improve the image quality of a 16-image series by two, a series of 64 images would be theoretically needed. Taking and processing (i.e., averaging) more images is not only more time-consuming and increases the exposure time to the patient's retina, but other practical restrictions may also occur, particularly in the case of unstable fixation. Before image averaging, single images must be aligned with each other to correct for eye movements during acquisition. This is performed by customized image analysis software, which is based on sophisticated algorithms to automatically match retinal landmarks between different images. The more images used for calculation of the mean image, the more complicated and difficult the alignment of the images to each other gets. This can result in poor alignment and, finally, in lower image quality, with fuzzy borders of retinal structures, than if a smaller number of images is used. Therefore, in most cases it is more practicable to use a reasonable number of single images to calculate the mean image (Fig. 4.1d).

A further development in modern cSLO systems includes the ability to obtain mean images during the acquisition process (so-called real-time averaging). This new feature for FAF images allows recording of FAF images in less time and marked reduction of the signal-to-noise ratio by averaging up to 100 images. This approach may be more practical, but it may lead to different results and has been not systematically compared with the usual image processing procedure.

4.4

Normalizing of FAF Image

Following the calculation of the mean image, the pixel values within the FAF image are usually normalized to better visualize the distribution of FAF intensities for the human eye (Fig. 4.1e). Although this final step facilitates the evaluation of intraindividual topographic differences and the interpretation of localized alterations of the signal in one image, it can make comparisons among different FAF images difficult. Pixel values of normalized images should be used only for a relative analysis (after taking differences of optical media and differences between acquisition settings into account). Absolute pixel values must not be used for the quantitative assessment of autofluorescence intensities between normalized FAF images. This important limitation is valid for comparing normalized FAF images between eyes as well as images of the same eye within longitudinal observations.

Furthermore, incorrect settings during the acquisition process, particularly with regard to the sensitivity of the detector, may not be seen on a normalized FAF image at first glance and may lead to false interpretations of FAF findings (Fig. 4.2e,f). Therefore, it is prudent to review single images as well.

Details within areas of markedly increased or decreased FAF signal intensity may also be obscured on images because of the normalizing algorithm. The software of modern cSLO imaging systems permits easy deactivation of the normalizing of mean images. Brightness and contrast can be manually adjusted on non-normalized mean images to better visualize the intensity distribution within such areas and to make more details visible for the human eye.

4.5
Standardized Protocol for FAF Imaging

- Adjust the chin rest and seat; the patient should be in a comfortable position.
- Start with near-infrared reflection mode and a frame size of 30°×30°.
- Set the focus of the optics roughly to the patient's spherical equivalent refraction.
- Ask the patient not to move his or her eyes, to fixate straight ahead, and to keep the eyes wide open.
- Move the camera toward the patient's eye by orienting the laser beam through the center of the pupils toward the macular area, and find the optimal camera-to-cornea distance.
- Refocus the image; adjust the sensitivity and laser power.
- The frame should encompass the entire macula area, with the fovea in the vertical center and the temporal part of the optic disc.
- Switch from near-infrared to blue-light (or so-called red-free) laser.
- Adjust the sensitivity and focus in blue-light reflectance mode (by decreasing refraction to correct for different chromatic aberrations between laser wavelengths).
- Set the barrier filter in front of the detector.
- Increase and adjust the sensitivity for FAF imaging.

- Acquire a movie of FAF images with a series of at least 15 single images, or acquire an averaged FAF image in real-time mode.

- Save images and exit acquisition mode.

- If FAF images are not acquired in real-time averaging mode, open the FAF image series and check each single image for eye movements or blinking.

- Delete single distorted or obscured images.

- Select the 12 best images for automatic alignment and calculation of a mean image (noting that more or fewer images sometimes lead to a better mean image).

4.6
Pitfalls

4.6.1
Focus

FAF image quality can be improved by optimal focusing for the blue-laser wavelength in the reflectance mode. Because of chromatic aberrations, the optimal refractive setting slightly differs between near-infrared and blue light, and the focus knob should be adjusted by decreasing the refractive power when switching from the near-infrared to the blue laser. This effect is shown in the following images: Reflectance images ("red-free mode") and final (averaged and normalized) FAF images are recorded directly after optimal focus adjustment in the infra-red mode (Fig. 4.2a,b). Image quality is slightly improved by better visualization of fine details after focus corrections for the blue-wavelength laser light (Fig. 4.2c,d).

4.6.2
Detector Sensitivity

False sensitivity adjustments of the detector can cause low image quality and may lead to inaccurate interpretation of FAF findings. In the case of a very low sensitivity setting during acquisition (underexposed), the contrast between retinal structures in the final normalized and averaged image is reduced (Fig. 4.2e). Note that because of the normalization of the pixel distribution, the actual image does not appear very dark. This could be seen only on a single image of this series. Without the examiner's awareness of this phenomenon, this artefact may not be recognized, and the analysis could lead to inadequate conclusions. Figure 4.2f illustrates the averaged and normalized image of a series of images that were clearly overexposed, caused by a too-high sensitivity setting of the detector during acquisition. Central foveal structures may appear slightly more visible, probably by partly overcoming macula pigment absorption. However, a meaningful analysis of FAF intensities outside the fovea is not possible.

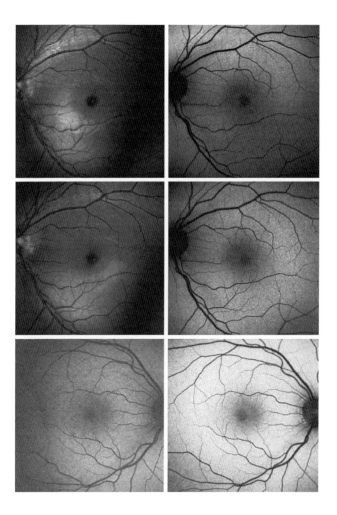

Fig. 4.2 Pitfalls—part 1. **a** *(top left)* Blue-light reflectance image immediately after adjusting the settings for near-infrared mode and without refocusing for shorter wavelength. **b** *(top right)* Normalized mean fundus autofluorescence (FAF) image with the same settings (out of focus). **c** *(middle left)* Blue-light reflectance image now refocused. **d** *(middle right)* Normalized mean FAF image with the same settings (in focus). **e** *(bottom left)* Normalized mean FAF image obtained from underexposed single images. **f** *(bottom right)* Normalized mean FAF image obtained from overexposed single images

4.6.3
Distance of Laser Scanning Camera to Cornea

An incorrect distance between the laser scanning camera and the cornea represents a common pitfall that leads to an obvious shadowing of the corners of the images. As both the blue-light reflectance (Fig. 4.3a) and the FAF (Fig. 4.3b) image illustrate this shadowing, it demonstrates that the low intensities at the corners of the FAF images are actually not a low autofluorescence signal of retinal structures, but clearly an artefact. To avoid this common pitfall, one should primarily ensure that the patient's head is firmly positioned on the chin and head rest and that the patient does not move backward during the acquisition. The optimal distance between camera and cornea should then be found—neither too close nor too far—until the corners of the image are optimally illuminated. A stable fixation and positioning in front of the camera may sometimes be difficult to achieve, particularly when taking FAF images and exposing a patient to the uncomfortable blue light for the first time. Under these circumstances, it may be helpful to get the patient somewhat accustomed to the blue light first. This can be achieved by moving the camera far back, switching the blue laser on, asking the patient to look straight ahead, and then slowly moving the camera toward the patient until the optimal distance is reached.

4.6.4
Illumination

Shadowing within an image is often an artefact and not actually caused by changes at the level of the retinal pigment epithelium (RPE). Irregular shadows are typically caused by vitreous opacities (see Fig. 4.4e), while very obvious shadows with common patterns affecting the whole image usually result from false settings during acquisition. The latter shadows typically follow a vertical or horizontal line through the image or—when caused by the wrong distance between camera and cornea (see previous section, 4.6.3)—are restricted to the corners of the images. An example of a vertical shadow in the temporal part of the images is illustrated in Fig. 4.3c. This shadow was caused by an incorrect positioning of the scan angle and can be easily adjusted by slightly moving the laser scanning camera nasally. To avoid uneven illuminations, it is important to identify these phenomena and to take sufficient time to find the optimal cSLO position before acquiring images.

4.6.5
Image Orientation

For assessment of FAF characteristics of the posterior pole, the image should encompass the macular area with the fovea in the vertical center and at least the temporal part of the optic nerve head. The latter is important as a retinal landmark and may facilitate the alignment process for the image analysis software, particularly in the presence of media opacities. Centering the image not only allows a reliable and meaningful analysis of FAF findings on a single examination, but it becomes even more important when FAF changes are compared over time. For example, to assess progression of atrophic patches in geographic atrophy over time, differences in the axial orientation of the laser scanner between individual examinations may cause slight distortions (see Fig. 12.2). Although these different angles can be corrected by aligning the images at different visits with image analysis software, they potentially still influence the accurate quantification of atrophic areas and may lead to incorrect measurements. Fig. 4.3d illustrates an extreme example in which the frame is not optimally centered at all. This decentering makes a meaningful analysis of FAF characteristics of the macula area practically impossible. To avoid such images, it is essential to ensure an optimal camera position. The comfortable positioning of the patient, including optimal height adjustment of the seat and chin rest, is an important prerequisite. If the patient does not look perfectly straight ahead, then first slightly move the chin rest up or down before turning the camera in extreme positions (i.e., directing the laser beam from far below or ahead). If the patient is cooperative and has good central visual function, instruct him or her to fixate at the center of the blue laser light that can be seen in the middle of the camera lens, or turn the fixation light on if available. The fixation light is blue and is therefore better recognized in the near-infrared mode. However, once the patient has fixated on the light in the near-infrared mode, he or she can usually still see it when switching to the blue laser light.

4.6.6

Eye Movements

Acquiring a series of FAF images for calculation of the mean image or acquiring FAF images with real-time averaging requires stable fixation. Before the calculation of the mean image (see Section 4.3), eye movements and blinking during the acquisition are corrected by aligning single images from a series. Depending on the patient's ability to keep the eyes in a stable position, the optimal number of single images for averaging can differ greatly among patients. Before selecting images for the averaging process, one should review every single image. Images with blinking or eye movements should be deleted and only good-quality images with similar frames marked. Figure 4.3e shows the result following averaging of 12 randomly selected images from one series with very instable fixation. The algorithms for image alignment could obviously not overlay the images correctly. However, after going back to the same series and carefully selecting eight good-quality images, a reasonable image quality of the final averaged and normalized image was achieved (Fig. 4.3f). This example demonstrates the importance of carefully selecting images and also illustrates that selecting fewer images can sometimes result in a better final image.

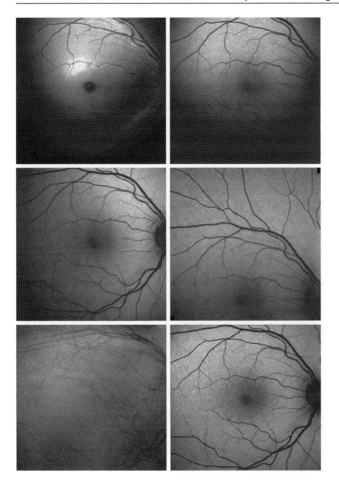

Fig. 4.3 Pitfalls—part 2. **a** *(top left)* Blue-light reflectance image with incorrect camera-to-cornea distance. **b** *(top right)* Fundus autofluorescence (FAF) image with the same settings (incorrect camera-to-cornea distance). **c** *(middle left)* FAF image with uneven illumination (incorrect axial laser scanner orientation). **d** *(middle right)* FAF image, not centered on fovea. **e** *(bottom left)* FAF image in the presence of unstable fixation. **f** *(bottom right)* FAF image calculated from eight single images from the same series as in the previous figure

4.7
Media Opacities

FAF image quality can be significantly impaired by opacities anterior to fluorescent lipofuscin granules in the RPE, at the level of the cornea, the anterior chamber, the lens, or the vitreous. Media opacities can also result in abnormal, nontypical distributions of FAF intensities in the form of irregular shadows. Confusion or even false interpretation of FAF findings may result. Clinical findings and the patient's history may give important clues to avoid this. To investigate unusual FAF phenomena and to differentiate between true alterations and artefacts, it is also helpful to look at the blue-light reflectance images and to compare them with the FAF images that were obtained with the same excitation wavelength. In the presence of media opacities, the incident light in front of retinal structures would be absorbed in both imaging modalities, with subsequent reduced emission and similar intensity distribution of the autofluorescence and the reflectance signal.

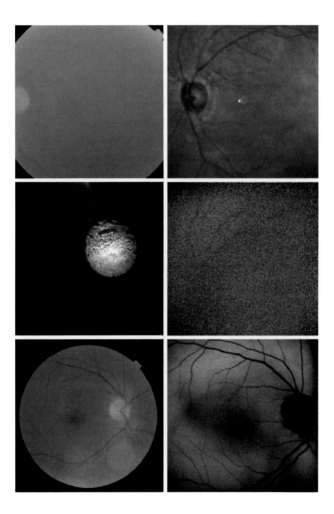

Fig. 4.4 Media opacities. Fundus photograph (**a,** *top left*), near-infrared reflectance (**b,** *top right*), blue-light reflectance (**c,** *middle left*), and fundus autofluorescence image (**d,** *middle right*) of the left eye of a patient with extreme yellowing of the lens in the absence of any obvious retinal abnormalities. Fundus photograph (**e,** *bottom left*) and fundus autofluorescence image (**f,** *bottom right*) of the right eye of a patient complaining of floaters.

The blue excitation light can be absorbed to a large extent by advanced cataract with nuclear sclerosis or advanced yellowing of the lens. Figure 4.4a–d illustrates fundus photograph and cSLO findings of the left eye of a patient with severe yellowing of the lens but with no known retinal abnormalities. Some details can still be seen on the fundus photograph (Fig. 4.4a). The near-infrared reflectance image demonstrates that reasonable (and better, compared with the fundus photograph) visualization of retinal structures is possible with the cSLO using a longer excitation wavelength (Fig. 4.4b). However, the absorption of the blue light by the yellow lens is so intense that hardly any retinal details are visible on either blue-light reflectance or FAF images (Fig. 4.4c, d). Note that the roundish structure on the reflectance image is caused by a reflection of the excitation light by the ocular media. This extreme example of insufficient FAF image quality caused by lens opacities illustrates the importance of blue-light reflectance images to identify artefacts.

Figure 4.4e and Fig. 4.4f illustrate fundus and FAF images of the right eye of a patient without retinal pathology. The patient had complained of severe floaters. The FAF image shows an irregular shadow in the center. This is not caused by absorption of irregular macula pigment distribution, but by absorption of vitreous opacities anterior to the retina.

References

1.   American National Standards Institute (2000) American national standard for the safe use of lasers: ANSI Z136.1. Laser Institute of America, Orlando, FL

2.   Schmitz-Valckenberg, S, Jorzik, J, Unnebrink, K, Holz, FG (2002) Analysis of digital scanning laser ophthalmoscopy fundus autofluorescence images of geographic atrophy in advanced age-related macular degeneration. Graefes Arch Clin Exp Ophthalmol 240:73–78

3.   von Rückmann, A, Fitzke, FW, Bird, AC (1995) Distribution of fundus autofluorescence with a scanning laser ophthalmoscope. Br J Ophthalmol 79:407–412

Autofluorescence Imaging with the Fundus Camera

5

Richard F. Spaide

5.1
Introduction

Autofluorescence photography provides functional images of the fundus by employing the stimulated emission of light from naturally occurring fluorophores, the most significant being lipofuscin. In the case of retinal pigment epithelial (RPE) cells, the build-up of lipofuscin is related in large part to the phagocytosis of photoreceptor outer segments containing damage accumulated through use; indigestible, altered molecules are retained within lysosomes and eventually become lipofuscin. Since the accumulation of lipofuscin occurs in RPE cells because of their unique metabolic role [1–3], autofluorescence imaging provides functional information about these cells.

One important component of lipofuscin in RPE cells is A2E [4]. There are fluorophores within the eye other than lipofuscin. Precursors of A2E, such as A2PE-H_2, A2PE, and A2-rhodopsin, all of which are autofluorescent, form in outer segments prior to phagocytosis by the RPE [5, 6]. There is no significant accumulation of the autofluorescent material within the retina unless a disease process exists that limits the RPE's ability to phagocytose the outer segments [7, 8]. If the anatomic relationship between the photoreceptor outer segments and the RPE is intact, the intensity of autofluorescence states parallels the amount and distribution of lipofuscin [9–11]. In cases in which there is a functional or spatial perturbation of the photoreceptor outer segment–RPE relationship, additional fluorophores can accumulate that are not, strictly speaking, lipofuscin, which is an intracellular accumulation of indigestible material within lysosomes.

5.2
Imaging Autofluorescence with a Fundus Camera

Lipofuscin can be made to fluoresce and has a broad emission band ranging from about 500 nm to 750 nm (Fig. 5.1) [9]. Directly illuminating the eye with excitation light will stimulate the lipofuscin, but other structures in the eye in front of the retina also fluoresce. The main culprit in this regard is the crystalline lens, which has a broad band of fluorescence principally from blue and green fluorophores that increase with age (see chapter 2.4). The fluorescent emission from the crystalline lens varies with the excitation light used, the age of the patient, the amount of nuclear sclerosis, and the concurrent diseases that may be present, such as diabetes. The lens fluorescence has a broad peak ranging from 500 to about 550 nm for the commonly used wavelengths for autofluorescence photography of the fundus. Therefore, autofluorescence of the crystalline lens overlaps the fluorescence produced by fluorescein. To produce useful autofluorescence images, we need to be able to either reject or bypass the fluorescence of the lens.

Scanning laser ophthalmoscopes have a confocal capability in which only conjugate points on the fundus are imaged. Points not lying on the conjugate planes are rejected. This allows confocal scanning laser ophthalmoscopes (cSLOs) to use excitation and barrier wavelengths similar to those used in fluorescein angiography to obtain autofluorescence photographs. Delori et al. used a 550 nm excitation filter with a glass-absorbing filter centered at 590 nm. The camera system used a charge-coupled-device camera cooled to −20°C and a restricted field of view of 13° "to minimize the loss in contrast caused by light scattering and fluorescence from the crystalline lens." This system was capable of imaging autofluorescence, but the published images had low contrast, and a 13° field of view is not acceptable for clinical practice [12].

Later development of a fundus-based camera system involved moving the excitation and emission wavelengths more toward the red end of the spectrum to avoid lens autofluorescence [13]. This was accomplished by using a band-pass filter centered at about 580 nm for excitation and one centered at about 695 nm as a barrier filter. The wavelengths used are not expected to show much attenuation from nuclear sclerosis. Because the lens fluorescence occurs with wavelengths shorter than the upper cutoff of the barrier filter, lens autofluorescence is usually not much of a problem unless the patient has severe degrees of nuclear sclerosis. The limitations of this system for autofluorescence include all of those that a typical fundus camera would face, particularly for patients with small pupils. Initial autofluorescent photography was possible with this system, but the signal was low, resulting in dark images. Increasing the gain, along with increasing the brightness of the photographs by normalizing the picture, increased the noise. The barrier filter was placed in the near-infrared region, which was on the far, declining edge of the fluorescence spectrum of lipofuscin. The optical performance of the camera and the eye is better adapted to visible wavelengths. Finally, longer wavelengths of light can penetrate through tissue to a greater extent than shorter wavelengths, so fluorescence originating from deeper levels of tissue can decrease the contrast of the images acquired from more proximal layers of interest.

To improve the image quality, a new set of filters was used in a fundus camera system. The excitation filter was selected to mimic the function of a green monochromatic filter by using a band-pass filter from 535 to 580 nm, which is not within the absorption curve of fluorescein; therefore, autofluorescence photography can be performed on a patient who has had fluorescein angiography. The wavelengths selected are not efficient at causing crystalline lens autofluorescence, a potential source of sig-

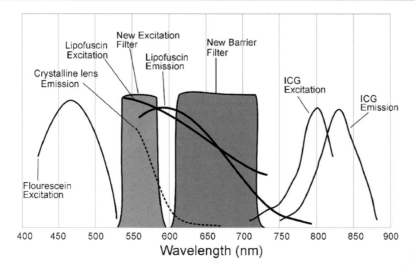

Fig. 5.1 Absorption and emission spectra involved in autofluorescence with the excitation and emission characteristics used in a newer version of fundus-camera-based autofluorescence photography. The crystalline lens fluorescence was not directly measured with this excitation filter but was extrapolated from published sources [14–18]. Note that the peak fluorescence from any given fluorophore, such as lipofuscin, depends on the excitation wavelength

nal degradation. The barrier filter is a band-pass filter transmitting from 615 nm to 715 nm. The separation in the filters affords a rejection of at least 10^{-7} of the excitation light coming from the fundus through the barrier filter. The barrier filter also blocks passage of longer-wavelength infrared light to avoid image degradation. The images are brighter, and there is less noise in the images than with earlier filters. There are numerous potential fluorophores in the fundus, with varying absorption and emission spectra. The differing wavelengths used by the cSLO and the fundus camera systems suggest that each system may record fluorescence from a somewhat dissimilar complement of fluorophores.

5.3
Differences Between the Autofluorescence Images Taken with a Fundus Camera and a cSLO

With the commercially available cSLO, 15 images are taken, and it is common for the best nine to be selected for image averaging because each individual image is weak and noisy. Because noise is generally a random event, whereas signal is not, averaging several images together causes the noise to be reduced proportionally to the square root of the number of images averaged (see chapter 4). In areas where there is a weak signal, averaging images with noise raises the mean grayscale level slightly. The commercially available cSLO then scales the image so that the histogram of the grayscale values better fits the available range, and in the process it appears to clip the black portion of the histogram. The statistical nature of how noise affects an image can lead to small variations in how regions of decreased autofluorescence, such as geographic atrophy, are imaged (Fig. 5.2). The wavelengths used by the commercially available cSLO are absorbed by nuclear sclerosis and macular pigment.

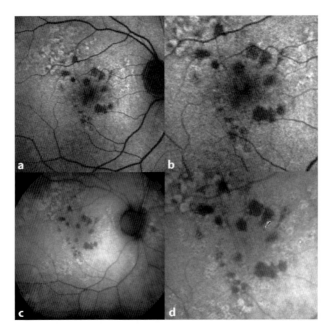

Fig. 5.2 Autofluorescent images taken of a patient with drusen and early geographic atrophy. **a** The commercially available confocal scanning laser ophthalmoscopy (cSLO) picture shows areas of hypoautofluorescence, including a butterfly-shaped area located in the central macula. **b** Enlargement of the central portion of image **a** to show the resolution and noise. Note that the vessels are easily seen because the wavelengths used for autofluorescence in the commercially available cSLO for autofluorescence are highly absorbed by hemoglobin. There were visible differences in the size of hypoautofluorescent regions among successively taken photographs. **c** A fundus camera picture of the same patient. Note the light falloff or vignetting toward the *edges* of the picture. The vessels do not display marked contrast because hemoglobin is relatively more transparent to the wavelengths used. **d** Enlargement of the central portion of image **c**, showing the relatively low noise of the image and the lack of effect of macular pigment on the autofluorescence detected. Note the ringlike autofluorescent changes around drusen, a feature seen because the retinal pigment epithelium is thinner on the surface of an individual druse and is thicker and seen in profile at the outer edges of the druse. This feature is lost in the noise for most of the drusen shown in image **b** (see also chapter 12.2)

The wavelengths used with the modified fundus camera are not absorbed as much by blood as compared with the wavelengths applied in the commercially available cSLO. This makes the contrast between the vessels and background less in fundus camera images than in the cSLO. This same factor may be a reason why the optic nerve often shows more fluorescence with a fundus camera system than with the cSLO. Fundus camera systems are inherently more affected by scattering than are cSLO methods of imaging. These factors may contribute to a reduced ability to discern smaller retinal vessels as compared with the cSLO. The wavelengths used in the fundus camera are not absorbed by macular pigment or fluorescein. Fundus cameras use a cone of light entering the eye around the region used for imaging. The intensity of autofluorescence is reduced by small pupillary apertures. Lens autofluorescence is prominent in patients with advanced degrees of nuclear sclerosis and needs to be manually removed from fundus camera images. The gradations in grayscale values in fundus camera images appear more smooth and capable of rendering subtle changes than a commercially available cSLO, probably because of reduced noise. The autofluorescent capabilities of the commercially available cSLO are built into the machine, as is the software. This is not yet true for fundus cameras, although autofluorescence filters are slated for inclusion in all new fundus cameras by at least one manufacturer.

References

1.   Eldred GE. Lipofuscin fluorophore inhibits lysosomal protein degradation and may cause early stages of macular degeneration. Gerontology 1995;41(Suppl 2):15–28

2.   Gaillard ER, Atherton SJ, Eldred G, Dillon J. Photophysical studies on human retinal lipofuscin. Photochem Photobiol 1995;61:448–453

3.   Li W, Yanoff M, Li Y, He Z. Artificial senescence of bovine retinal pigment epithelial cells induced by near-ultraviolet in vitro. Mech Ageing Dev 1999 22;110:137–155

4.   Reinboth JJ, Gautschi K, Munz K, Eldred GE, Reme CE. Lipofuscin in the retina: quantitative assay for an unprecedented autofluorescent compound (pyridinium bis-retinoid, A2-E) of ocular age pigment. Exp Eye Res 1997;65:639–643

5.   Liu J, Itagaki Y, Ben-Shabat S, Nakanishi K, Sparrow JR. The biosynthesis of A2E, a fluorophore of aging retina, involves the formation of the precursor, A2-PE, in the photoreceptor outer segment membrane. J Biol Chem 2000 22;275:29354–29360

6.   Fishkin N, Jang YP, Itagaki Y, et al. A2-rhodopsin: a new fluorophore isolated from photoreceptor outer segments. Org Biomol Chem 2003 7;1:1101–1105

7.   Spaide RF, Klancnik Jr JM. Fundus autofluorescence and central serous chorioretinopathy. Ophthalmology 2005;112:825–833

8.   Spaide RF, Noble K, Morgan A, Freund KB. Vitelliform macular dystrophy. Ophthalmology 2006;113:1392–1400

9.   Delori FC, Dorey CK, Staurenghi G, et al. In vivo fluorescence of the ocular fundus ex-
     hibits retinal pigment epithelium lipofuscin characteristics. Invest Ophthalmol Vis Sci
     1995;36:718–729

10. Wing GL, Blanchard GC, Weiter JJ. The topography and age relationship of lipofuscin con-
     centration in the retinal pigment epithelium. Invest Ophthalmol Vis Sci 1978;17:601–607

11. von Ruckmann A, Fitzke FW, Bird AC. Distribution of fundus autofluorescence with a scan-
     ning laser ophthalmoscope. Br J Ophthalmol 1995;79:407–412

12. Delori FC, Fleckner MR, Goger DG, et al. Autofluorescence distribution associated with
     drusen in age-related macular degeneration. Invest Ophthalmol Vis Sci 2000;41:496–504

13. Spaide RF. Fundus autofluorescence and age-related macular degeneration. Ophthalmology
     2003;110:392–399

14. Eldred GE, Katz ML. Fluorophores of the human retinal pigment epithelium: separation and
     spectral characterization. Exp Eye Res 1988;47:71–86

15. Rozanowska M, Pawlak A, Rozanowski B, et al. Age-related changes in the photoreactivity
     of retinal lipofuscin granules: role of chloroform-insoluble components. Invest Ophthalmol
     Vis Sci. 2004;45:1052–1060

16. Haralampus-Grynaviski NM, Lamb LE, Clancy CM, et al. Spectroscopic and morphological
     studies of human retinal lipofuscin granules. Proc Natl Acad Sci USA. 2003;100:3179–3184

17. Pawlak A, Rozanowska M, Zareba M, et al. Action spectra for the photoconsumption of
     oxygen by human ocular lipofuscin and lipofuscin extracts. Arch Biochem Biophys.
     2002;403:59–62

18. Marmorstein AD, Marmorstein LY, Sakaguchi H, Hollyfield JG. Spectral profiling of auto-
     fluorescence associated with lipofuscin, Bruch's membrane, and sub-RPE deposits in normal
     and AMD eyes. Invest Ophthalmol Vis Sci 2002;43:2435–2441

Macular Pigment Measurement— Theoretical Background

Sebastian Wolf, Ute E.K. Wolf-Schnurrbusch

6.1
Introduction

Age-related macular degeneration (AMD) is the leading cause of visual loss in the industrialised world for people over 65 years of age [6, 7]. Although the exact pathophysiology of AMD remains poorly understood, there is growing evidence that the development of age-related maculopathy is related to oxidative damage [8, 11, 30]. Because many antioxidative properties are attributed to the macular pigment, it has been investigated with respect to its role in the pathological concept of AMD [23–25]. The first investigations on the function of macular pigment were performed by Max Schultze, who concluded in 1866 that there is a functional connection between the "yellow spot" in the retina and the absorption of blue light.

6.2
Functional and Physiological Properties of Macular Pigment

The macular pigment consists of the two hydroxy carotenoids lutein and zeaxanthin. Lutein and zeaxanthin reach their highest concentration in the centre of the fovea. Zeaxanthin is the leading carotenoid in this location. With increasing eccentricity, zeaxanthin values decline more rapidly than lutein values, leading to lutein being the main carotenoid in the peripheral locations. The zeaxanthin/lutein ratio changes with eccentricity in favour of lutein [5, 26]. Optically undetectable levels are reached at an eccentricity of 1.2–1.5 mm from the foveal centre [17, 26]. By means of high-performance liquid chromatography (HPLC), carotenoids are detectable in the whole retina [18].

In primates, carotenoids cannot be synthesised de novo and have to be taken in by nutrition. Hammond et al. analysed the correlation between dietary intake of xanthophylls, blood serum levels, and macular pigment density in humans and found a positive relationship between these factors [16]. This variability of the macular pigment initiated by nutritional supplementation makes it an interesting target for future intervention, with the aim to prevent or alter the course of AMD.

The role of macular pigment includes a high capacity to absorb short-wavelength blue light. This could be named a passive protection mode [24]. The peak of the macular pigment absorbance spectrum is at 460 nm and works as a broad band filter for the macula. Two advantages are achieved: the macula's optical accuracy is improved [10, 17], and the damaging photo-oxidative influence on the neurosensory retina is reduced. Ham et al. showed that the threshold for retinal damage induced by different wavelengths of light fell exponentially with decreasing wavelength [15].

The macular pigment's ability as a blue-light filter has four basic features. The absorbance spectrum of macular pigment peaks at 460 nm. In addition, the highest carotenoid concentration is in the pre-receptoral axon layer of the fovea and the extrafoveal macula. This enables the macular pigment in the fovea to reach a high proportion of absorption before the light can cause its damaging effect on the photoreceptors.

In the photoreceptor outer segments, the antioxidant effect of lutein and zeaxanthin is the essential mechanism. The antioxidant properties enable the carotenoids to neutralise free radicals, which are partially reduced oxygen species with one or more unpaired electrons. These belong to a group of so-called reactive oxygen species (ROS); they all have in common high reactivity with lipid, protein, and nucleic acids, leading to cell damage or death [14]. A factor leading to a high retinal sensitivity to oxidative influence is the combination of light exposure and high oxygen levels. This provides an ideal environment for the generation of ROS and a high concentration of unsaturated fatty acids. Carotenoids protect membrane lipids from toxic peroxidation, and macular pigment is sometimes called a free-radical scavenger [1].

Another feature is related to the filtering effect of blue light and thus the reduction of one of the two components that leads to the generation of ROS. Relatively high concentrations of oxidative carotenoid metabolites indicate that they might be a product of antioxidative activity [22].

6.3
Detection of Macular Pigment

Snodderly examined the macular pigment density of macaque and squirrel monkeys by means of microdensitometry and HPLC [26]. Bone et al. used reversed-phase HPLC to quantify retinal lutein and zeaxanthin in relation to an internal standard. They analysed donor-eye retinas from subjects with and without AMD. There appeared to be a significant higher concentration of lutein and zeaxanthin in eyes without AMD than in those with AMD [5]. The results imply an inverse association between the risk of AMD and macular pigment density.

Heterochromatic flicker photometry is a widely used psychophysical technique. The patient seeks to eliminate flicker in a visual stimulus that alternates between two wavelengths. These are usually chosen from the blue (460 nm, wavelength of absorbance maximum) and green (540 nm, absorption essentially zero) portions of the spectrum. Although this method is relatively easy to apply, it is dependent on the patient's compliance and the condition of the macula. Patients with macular pathologies such as advanced-stage AMD may find it difficult to complete the examination.

The group of Bone et al. published a study in which the relationship between dietary intake of lutein and zeaxanthin, blood serum levels of lutein and zeaxanthin, and the optical density of macular pigment were analysed [4]. About 30% of the variability of the macular pigment density could be attributed to the serum concentration of lutein and zeaxanthin.

Ciulla et al. utilised heterochromatic flicker photometry to measure macular pigment before and after cataract extraction and found that differences in retinal illuminance due to varying opaqueness of the crystalline lens have no measurable influence on macular pigment optical density [9].

In 1998 Bernstein et al. introduced an objective method to measure macular pigment in post-mortem human retinas and in experimental animal eyes [3]. It is based on a Raman spectrometer, which detects retinal signals that are a reaction to argon laser excitation. The results are promising, indicating that the Raman signals achieved from human post-mortem retinas match those achieved in standardised lutein solutions.

Elsner et al. compared the distribution of cone photo pigment and macular pigment of healthy subjects before the age of possible onset of AMD [13]. The macular pigment was measured by reflectometry using a scanning laser ophthalmoscope (SLO) with 488 nm and 514 nm light illumination.

Berendschot et al. used the SLO to measure macular pigment density as well [2]. The results were compared with those obtained by the foveal fundus reflectance measured with a fundus reflectometer. Besides assessment of the quality of the new method, the second aim of this study was to evaluate the benefit of nutritional carotenoid supplementation on macular pigment density. The results show high reliability of the SLO measurements, with fewer disturbing noises in the measurements compared with spectral analysis. SLO measurements showed a substantial and significant increase in macular pigment density in the course of dietary supplementation with carotenoids and also a significant correlation between plasma lutein levels and macular pigment density as determined with both macular pigment maps and spectral analysis.

A new approach to in-vivo measurements has been introduced by Delori et al. [12]. The detection of the autofluorescence of lipofuscin as activated by two wavelengths, one well absorbed by macular pigment and one minimally absorbed, enables the examiner to obtain accurate single-pass measurements of the macular pigment density. The results seem to highly correlate with the results taken from an alternative psychophysical method (heterochromatic flicker photometry) and another optic method (fundus reflectometry).

6.4
Measurement of Macular Pigment Density Using a cSLO

Based on the pioneering work of Delori [12], a clinical routine method was developed using a modified SLO (Fig. 6.1, mpHRA; Heidelberg Engineering, Heidelberg, Germany) for measuring macular pigment density [28]. This instrument is optimised to record autofluorescence images at 488 nm and 514 nm wavelengths. Because the absorption of macular pigment at 488 nm wavelength is very high and at 514 nm wavelength is close to zero, we can determine macular pigment density by comparing foveal and parafoveal reflectance at 488 nm and 514 nm (Fig. 6.2). For easy assessment of macular pigment density, density maps are calculated by digital subtraction of the log autofluorescence images (Fig. 6.3). Because the difference in absorption by pigments other than macular pigment (e.g. retinal and choroidal blood, visual pigments, retinal pigment epithelium, and choroidal melanin) between the fovea and 7° outside the fovea can be neglected, macular pigment density can be determined by comparing foveal and parafoveal autofluorescence. Various studies have demonstrated that this method leads to reliable and clinically relevant measurement of macular pigment [19–21, 27, 29].

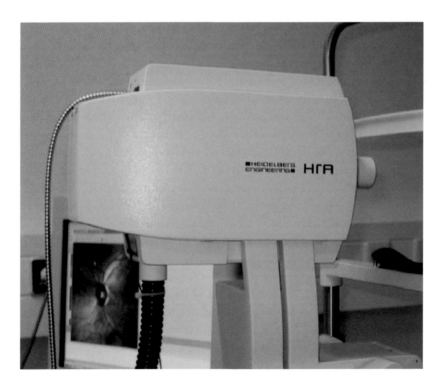

Fig. 6.1 Modified confocal scanning laser ophthalmoscope for macular pigment measurement

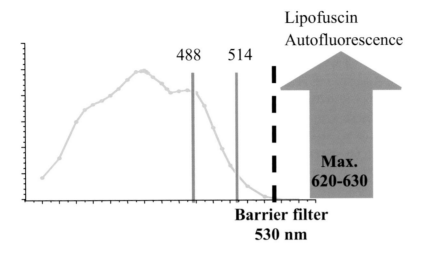

Fig. 6.2 Absorbance spectrum of macular pigment for visible light

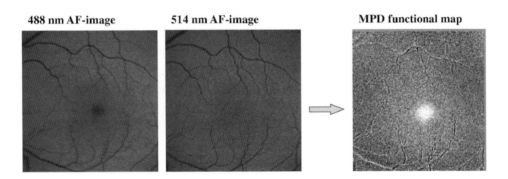

Fig. 6.3 Autofluorescence images taken at 488 nm and 514 nm wavelengths and the corresponding macular pigment density map calculated by digital subtraction of the autofluorescence images

References

1. Beatty S, Boulton M, Henson D, Koh HH, Murray IJ (1999) Macular pigment and age related macular degeneration. Br J Ophthalmol 83(7):867–877

2. Berendschot TT, Goldbohm RA, Klopping WA, van de Kraats J, van Norel J, van Norren D (2000) Influence of lutein supplementation on macular pigment, assessed with two objective techniques. Invest Ophthalmol Vis Sci 41(11):3322–3326

3. Bernstein PS, Yoshida MD, Katz NB, McClane RW, Gellermann W (1998) Raman detection of macular carotenoid pigments in intact human retina. Invest Ophthalmol Vis Sci 39:2003–2011

4. Bone RA, Landrum JT, Cains A (1992) Optical density spectra of the macular pigment in vivo and in vitro. Vision Res 32(1):105–110

5. Bone RA, Landrum JT, Fernandez lutein, Tarsis SL (1988) Analysis of the macular pigment by HPLC: retinal distribution and age study. Invest Ophthalmol Vis Sci 29(6):843–849

6. Bressler NM, Bressler SB (1995) Preventative ophthalmology age-related macular degeneration. Ophthalmology 102:1206–1211

7. Bressler NM, Bressler SB, West SK, Fine SL, Taylor HR (1989) The grading and prevalence of macular degeneration in Chesapeake Bay watermen. Arch Ophthalmol 107:847–852

8. Challa JK, Gillies MC, Penfold PL (1998) Exudative degeneration and intravitreal triamcinolone: 18 month follow up. Aust N zeaxanthin J Ophthalmol 26:277–281

9. Ciulla TA, Hammond BR, Jr., Yung CW, Pratt LM (2001) Macular pigment optical density before and after cataract extraction. Invest Ophthalmol Vis Sci 42(6):1338–1341

10. Dagnelie G, Zorge IS, McDonald TM (2000) Lutein improves visual function in some patients with retina degeneration: a pilot study via the internet. Optometry 71:147–164

11. De La Paz MA, Anderson RE (1992) Lipid peroxidation in rod outer segments. Role of hydroxyl and lipid hydroperoxides. Invest Ophthalmol Vis Sci 33:2091–2096

12. Delori FC, Goger DG, Hammond BR, Snodderly DM, Burns SA (2001) Macular pigment density measured by autofluorescence spectrometry: comparison with reflectometry and heterochromatic flicker photometry. J Opts Soc Am 18:1212–1230

13. Elsner AE, Burns SA, Huges GW, Webb RH (1992) Quantitative reflectometry with a scanning laser ophthalmoscope. Applied Optics 31(19):3697–3710

14. Halliwell B (1997) Antioxidants: the basics—what they are and how to evaluate them. Adv Pharmacol 38:3–20

15. Ham WTJ, Mueller HA, Sliney DH (1976) Retinal sensitivity to damage from short wavelength light. Nature 260:153–155

16. Hammond BR, Jr., Wooten BR, Snodderly DM (1996) Cigarette smoking and retinal carotenoids: implications for age-related macular degeneration. Vision Res 36(18):3003–3009

17. Hammond BR, Jr., Wooten BR, Snodderly DM (1997) Density of the human crystalline lens is related to the macular pigment carotenoids, lutein and zeaxanthin. Optom Vis Sci 74(7):499–504

18. Handelmann GJ, Dratz EA, Reay CC, van Kuijk JG (1988) Carotenoids in the human macula and whole retina. Invest Ophthalmol Vis Sci 29:850–855

19. Jahn C, Brinkmann C, Mößner A, Wüstemeyer H, Schnurrbusch U, Wolf S (2006) [Seasonal fluctuations and influence of nutrition on macular pigment density.] Der Ophthalmologe 103(2):136–140

20. Jahn C, Wüstemeyer H, Brinkmann C, Trautmann S, Mößner A, Schnurrbusch U, Wolf S (2004) Macular pigment densitiy subject to different stages of age-related maculopathy: ARVO abstract

21. Jahn C, Wustemeyer H, Brinkmann C, Trautmann S, Mossner A, Wolf S (2005) Macular pigment density in age-related maculopathy. Graefes Arch Clin Exp Ophthalmol 243(3):222–227

22. Khachik F, Bernstein PS, Garland DL (1997) Identification of lutein and zeaxanthin oxidation products in and monkey retinas. Invest Ophthalmol Vis Sci 38:1802–1811

23. Landrum JT, Bone RA (2001) Lutein, zeaxanthin, and the macular pigment. Arch Biochem Biophys 385(1):28–40

24. Landrum JT, Bone RA, Joa H, Kilburn MD, Moore LL, Sprague KE (1997) A one year study of the macular pigment: the effect of 140 days of a lutein supplement. Exp Eye Res 65(1):57–62

25. Snodderly DM (1995) Evidence for protection against age-related macular degeneration by carotenoids and antioxidant vitamins. Am J Clin Nutr 62(6 suppl):1448S–1461S

26. Snodderly DM, Handelman GJ, Adler AJ (1991) Distribution of individual macular pigment carotenoids in central retina of macaque and squirrel monkeys. Invest Ophthalmol Vis Sci 32(2):268–279

27. Trieschmann M, Beatty S, Nolan JM, Hense HW, Heimes B, Austermann U, Fobker M, Pauleikhoff D (2007) Changes in macular pigment optical density and serum concentrations of its constituent carotenoids following supplemental lutein and zeaxanthin: the LUNA study. Exp Eye Res 84(4):718–728

28. Wüstemeyer H, Jahn C, Nestler A, Barth T, Wolf S (2002) A new instrument for the quantification of macular pigment density: first results in patients with AMD and healthy subjects. Graefes Arch Clin Exp Ophthalmol 240(8):666–671

29. Wüstemeyer H, Mößner A, Jahn C, Wolf S (2003) Macular pigment densitiy in patients with ARM quantified with a modified confocal scanning laser. ophthalmoscope (ARVO abstract 2003)

30. Young RW (1987) Pathophysiology of age-related macular degeneration. Surv Ophthalmol 31:291–306

Macular Pigment Measurement — Clinical Applications

7

Frederik J.G.M. van Kuijk, Daniel Pauleikhoff

7.1
Introduction

Chapter 6 outlined various studies that have utilized autofluorescence imaging to measure macular pigment (MP) [14, 21, 22]. In addition to peak optical density, the autofluorescence method allows assessment of the shape of MP spatial distribution. There is considerable intersubject differences in MP spatial profiles, as recognized by several investigators [6, 7, 11, 14]. It is perhaps surprising that so many studies on MP, including some of those based on fundus imaging, focused solely on the peak optical density at the fovea and ignored the lateral distribution [3, 4, 21, 22]. A possible role for MP in the pathophysiology of age-related macular degeneration (AMD) has been suggested [2, 5], and Trieschmann et al. have reported that this can be related to the MP profiles [19].

7.2
Variability of Macula Pigment Distribution

Intersubject differences in MP distribution profiles have been documented using the established psychophysical technique of motion photometry [7, 14]. The lateral extent of MP distribution and the computed total complement of MP cannot be predicted from the peak optical density at the fovea [14]. An example is shown in Fig. 7.1, in which two subjects have similar peak MP optical density but different MP profiles. This underscores the importance of quantifying MP distribution rather than MP peak optical density alone when studies are performed regarding the role of MP in AMD. Calibrated grey-scale measurements of autofluorescence correlate with psychophysically derived MP optical density values [13]. The advantages of the autofluorescence method are that the peak MP optical density, spatial profile, and radial symmetry may be extracted from a single image and that the method is rapid and objective. Psychophysical methods are time-consuming and might typically take about 30 min to obtain a detailed spatial profile along a single axis. In addition, psychophysical testing may be demanding or impossible for the subject, particularly if vision is impaired. MP profiles can be estimated with single wavelength autofluorescence (Fig. 7.2), but there are limitations, as acknowledged in earlier studies [13, 14]. The underlying fluorophore may not have a uniform distribution and quantification is inevitably influenced by illumination gradients and optical artifacts. Trieschmann et al. compared single- and two-wavelength methods and suggested that single-wavelength autofluorescence, obtained using the widely available standard Heidelberg Retina Angiograph (HRA), would be a suitable screening tool in multicenter studies but that the two-wavelength method (Fig 7.3) was likely to provide a more precise assessment [18]. In addition, a recent histological study of 11 donor eyes showed significant differences in the spatial extent of luteal pigment across the macula [20].

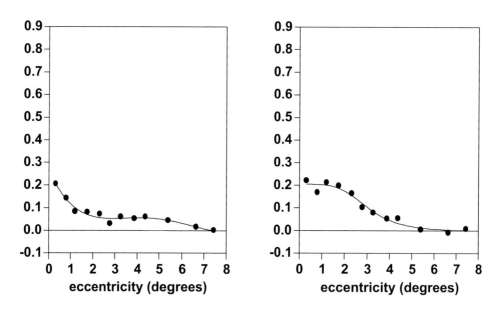

Fig. 7.1 Interindividual variation of macular pigment profiles. Note that both subjects have a similar peak optical density but variable amounts of macular pigment (part of a figure previously reported by Robson et al. [14])

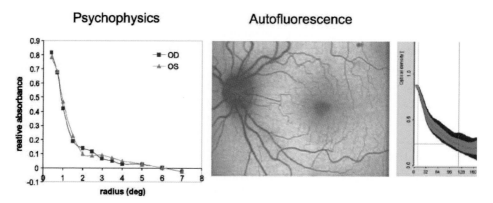

Fig. 7.2 Comparison of macular pigment distribution profile obtained by motion photometry and by autofluorescence. It is much faster to use the autofluorescence method. The minimum motion profile on the left is courtesy of Professor J.D. Moreland and Dr. A.G. Robson

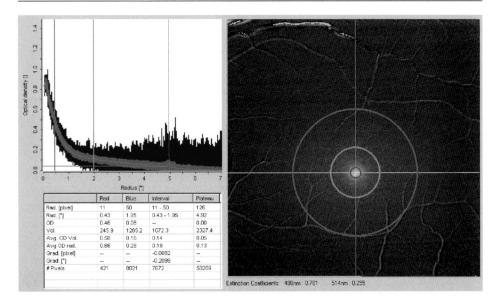

	Red	Blue	Interval	Plateau
Rad. [pixel]	11	50	11 - 50	126
Rad. [°]	0.43	1.95	0.43 - 1.95	4.92
OD	0.46	0.08	--	0.00
Vol.	245.9	1285.2	1072.3	2327.4
Avg. OD Vol.	0.58	0.16	0.14	0.05
Avg OD rad.	0.66	0.28	0.18	0.13
Grad. [pixel]	--	--	-0.0082	--
Grad. [°]	--	--	-0.2099	--
# Pixels	421	8021	7672	50269

Extinction Coefficients: 488nm : 0.781   514nm : 0.255

Fig. 7.3 Macular pigment (MP) density map calculated by digital subtraction of the autofluorescence images taken at 488 nm and 514 nm (see Chap. 6.4). Optical density can be obtained at various locations, as indicated by the *red, blue,* and *green circles.* The MP distribution profile shown on the left was obtained by obtaining optical density at each location

7.3
Genetic and Environmental Factors of Macular Pigment Distribution

There is a positive correlation between dietary intake of xanthophylls, blood serum levels, and peak MP optical density [8, 12]. Furthermore, Seddon et al. reported that dietary intake of macular carotenoids decreases risk for the development of exudative AMD [16]. This relationship of the MP optical density and AMD initiated by nutritional supplementation makes it an interesting target for future studies such as the Age-Related Eye Disease Study (AREDS) II, with the aim of preventing or altering the course of AMD. AREDS II is similar in design as the AREDS I study [1] but will additionally examine the influence of dietary lutein. Since most previous studies are based on peak MP optical density and not on MP spatial distribution, Liew et al. [10] examined genetic factors in a study with 150 twins, 76 monozygotic (MZ) and 74 dizygotic (DZ). MP spatial distribution profiles were measured with the two-wavelength autofluorescence method. The covariance of MP within MZ and DZ twin pairs was compared, and genetic modeling techniques were used to determine the relative contributions of genes and environment to the variation in MP. MP optical density profiles correlated more highly in MZ twins than in DZ twins, and the study demonstrated that genetic background is an important determinant of the MP optical density profile [10]. Figure 7.4 shows an example of MP optical density profiles of MZ and DZ twins.

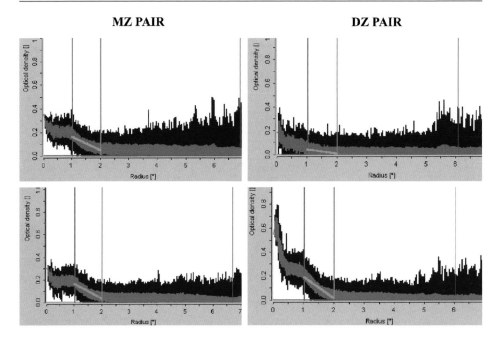

MZ PAIR   **DZ PAIR**

Fig. 7.4 Macular pigment optical density profiles of monozygotic (MZ) and dizygotic (DZ) twins. The profiles of the MZ siblings are almost identical, whereas the profiles of the DZ siblings are highly variable. Reprinted with permission

It is an interesting observation that the MP profiles may have a genetic background, especially if the MP spatial profile is more strongly related to AMD than the MP optical density [19]. Berendschot et al. [4] did not find a relationship between AMD and MP optical density. The question remains whether the MP spatial profile can be altered with supplements in a way so that the MP profile is modified enough to reduce the risk for AMD progression.

7.4
Macular Pigment Distribution: Effect of Supplementation

Early xanthophyll supplementation studies examined peak MP levels using the psychophysical technique of heterochromatic flicker photometry. In 1997 Landrum et al. presented data on supplementation of two subjects with a high dose of lutein (30 mg) for several months [9]. An increase in MP optical density was observed. Subsequently, Berendschot et al. [3] used scanning laser ophthalmoscopy to measure MP optical density after lower-dose (10 mg) carotenoid supplementation on MP density.

They showed a substantial and significant increase of MP optical density in the course of dietary supplementation with carotenoids. It should be noted that these and other studies did not involve randomization of the subjects and that in some cases the investigators were the subjects who were supplemented.

Several studies have been conducted using large numbers of subjects. The LUXEA (*LU*tein *X*anthophyll *E*ye *A*ccumulation) study was a double-blind controlled randomized trial in which MP was monitored using flicker photometry [15]. Dietary supplements of 10–20 mg of lutein (L) or zeaxanthin (Z) or a combination of the two were given for minimum periods of 6–12 months. MP optical density increased by 15% with L or L+Z supplementation. Psychophysical data suggested that supplementation with Z alone resulted in similar pigment accumulation in fovea and parafovea, which confounded standard computations of peak MP optical density relative to the parafovea [15]. After correction for this, a 14% MP optical density increase resulted for Z. Thus, during supplementation with xanthophylls, L is predominantly deposited in the fovea while Z deposition appears to cover a wider retinal area. This may be relevant to health and disease of the retina [15]. It should be noted that the study population consisted of healthy young males with baseline peak MP optical density values ranging from 0.20 to 0.70.

The LUNA (*LU*tein *N*utrition Effects Measured by *A*utofluorescence) study looked at 108 subjects supplemented with a formulation of L+Z esters in an 11:1 ratio [17]. It was found that there was a group of nonresponders and that the subjects with the lowest baseline MP optical density values had the highest likelihood of MP increases. Interestingly, there was also a considerable increase of MP optical density in the control group [17]. This may have been due to increasing awareness of dietary nutrition effects when consenting individuals participated.

7.5
Summary

The relationship between MP and AMD may depend on both the MP optical density and MP lateral distribution. The MP optical density profile may have a strong genetic background, and this profile is not easily altered with nutritional supplements. The AREDS II study is designed to determine whether lutein supplementation can reduce the risk of AMD progression.

Acknowledgements

The authors thank Professor Jack D. Moreland and Dr. Anthony G. Robson for motion photometry figures. We also appreciate comments on the manuscript by Dr. Anthony G. Robson.

References

1.   AREDS (1999) The Age-Related Eye Disease Study (AREDS): design implications AREDS report no. 1. The Age-Related Eye Disease Study Research Group. Control Clin Trials 20:573–600

2.   Beatty S, Murray IJ, Henson DB, et al. (2001) Macular pigment and risk for age-related macular degeneration in subjects from a Northern European population. Invest Ophthalmol Vis Sci 42:439–446

3.   Berendschot TT, Goldbohm RA, Klopping WA, et al. (2000) Influence of lutein supplementation on macular pigment, assessed with two objective techniques. Invest Ophthalmol Vis Sci 41:3322–3326

4.   Berendschot TT, Willemse-Assink JJ, Bastiaanse M, et al (2002) Macular pigment and melanin in age-related maculopathy in a general population. Invest Ophthalmol Vis Sci 43:1928–1932

5.   Bone RA, Landrum JT, Mayne ST, et al (2001) Macular pigment in donor eyes with and without AMD: a case-control study. Invest Ophthalmol Vis Sci 42:235–240

6.   Chen SF, Chang Y, Wu JC (2001) The spatial distribution of macular pigment in humans. Curr Eye Res 23:422–434

7.   Hammond BR, Wooten BR, Snodderly DM (1997) Individual variations in the spatial profile of human macular pigment. J Opt Soc Am A 14:1187–1196

8.   Johnson EJ, Hammond BR, Yeum K-J, et al (2000) Relation among serum and tissue concentrations of lutein and zeaxanthin and macular pigment density. Am J Clin Nutr 71:1555–1562

9.   Landrum JT, Bone RA, Joa H, Kilburn MD, Moore LL, Sprague KE (1997) A one year study of the macular pigment: the effect of 140 days of a lutein supplement. Exp Eye Res 65:57–62

10. Liew SH, Gilbert CE, Spector TD, et al (2005) Heritability of macular pigment: a twin study. Invest Ophthalmol Vis Sci 46:4430–4436

11. Moreland JD, Bhatt P (1984) Retinal distribution of macular pigment. In: Verriest G, Junck W. Colour vision deficiencies VII. Boston Lancastere, The Hague

12. Nolan JM, Stack J, O'connell E, et al (2007) The relationships between macular pigment optical density and its constituent carotenoids in diet and serum. Invest Ophthalmol Vis Sci 48:571–582

13. Robson AG, Harding G, Van Kuijk FJ, et al (2005) Comparison of fundus autofluorescence and minimum-motion measurements of macular pigment distribution profiles derived from identical retinal areas. Perception 34:1029–1034

14. Robson AG, Moreland JD, Pauleikhoff D, et al (2003) Macular pigment density and distribution: comparison of fundus autofluorescence with minimum motion photometry. Vis Res 43:1765–1775

15. Schalch W, Cohn W, Barker FM, et al (2007) Xanthophyll accumulation in the human retina during supplementation with lutein or zeaxanthin—the LUXEA (LUtein Xanthophyll Eye Accumulation) study. Arch Biochem Biophys 458:128–135

16. Seddon JM, Ajani UA, Sperduto RD, et al (1994) Dietary carotenoids, vitamins A, C, and E, and advanced age-related macular degeneration. JAMA 272:1413–1420

17. Trieschmann M, Beatty S, Nolan JM, et al (2007) Changes in macular pigment optical density and serum concentrations of its constituent carotenoids following supplemental lutein and zeaxanthin: the LUNA study. Exp Eye Res 84:718–728

18. Trieschmann M, Heimes B, Hense HW, et al (2006) Macular pigment optical density measurement in autofluorescence imaging: comparison of one- and two-wavelength methods. Graefes Arch Clin Exp Ophthalmol Apr 27 [Epub ahead of print]

19. Trieschmann M, Spital G, Lommatzsch A, et al (2003) Macular pigment: quantitative analysis on autofluorescence images. Graefes Arch Clin Exp Ophthalmol 241(12):1006–1012

20. Trieschmann M, Van Kuijk FJ, Alexander R, et al (2007) Macular pigment in the human retina: histological evaluation of localization and distribution. Eye (in press)

21. Wolf S, Brinkmann CK, Moessner A, et al (2003) Test-retest reproducibility of macular pigment density in healthy subjects quantified with a modified confocal scanning laser ophthalmoscope. Invest Ophthalmol Vis Sci 44:U217

22. Wustemeyer H, Moessner A, Jahn C, et al (2003) Macular pigment density in healthy subjects quantified with a modified confocal scanning laser ophthalmoscope. Graefes Arch Clin Exp Ophthalmol 241:647–651

Evaluation of Fundus Autofluorescence Images

Frank G. Holz, Monika Fleckenstein,
Steffen Schmitz-Valckenberg, Alan C. Bird

8

When a fundus autofluorescence (FAF) image is being evaluated, any deviation from a normal recording should be recognized, and a potential cause should be sought for the abnormal findings. The characteristics of a FAF image without disease-related abnormalities include the following (see Fig. 8.1, top row):

The **optic nerve head** typically appears dark because of the absence of retinal pigment epithelium (RPE) and, thus, autofluorescent lipofuscin.

The **retinal vessels** are associated with a markedly reduced FAF signal because of absorption phenomena from blood contents.

In the **macular area**, the FAF signal is most prominently reduced at the fovea. From the foveal center, a distinct increase in the signal can be observed at about the margin of the fovea, followed by a further gradual increment toward the outer macula. This is caused by absorption from luteal pigment (i.e., lutein and zeaxanthin) in the neurosensory retina and possible spatial differences in melanin deposition (see chapter 2). There is marked interindividual variation with regard to the topographic distribution of luteal pigment (see Chaps. 6 and 7).

Outside these areas with decrements in FAF intensity, the FAF signal appears evenly distributed. Advances in the optical and software development for the confocal scanning laser ophthalmoscope (cSLO) technique now even allow for delineation of the polygonal RPE-cell monolayer in the presence of clear media and optimal patient cooperation (Fig. 8.1, middle row). This delineation is possibly due to the spatial orientation of the lipofuscin and melanin granules in the RPE cell cytoplasm (see Fig. 8.1, bottom row). While there is typically a predominant location of lipofuscin granules at the peripheral cell margin, absorbing melanin granules are oriented toward the apical cell center.

Identification of abnormalities in the FAF image is very much dependent on the quality of the recorded image (see Chap. 4). Any opacities in the vitreous, the lens, the anterior chamber, or the cornea may affect the detection of pathological alterations at the level of the RPE and the neurosensory retina. Lens opacities particularly have an impact on the image quality, with yellowish alterations of the nucleus with age leading to absorption of the blue excitation light used for FAF imaging. Images recorded with fundus cameras using equivalent filters are affected more by such lens changes compared with recordings from cSLOs. However, in the presence of advanced lenticular changes, it may be impossible to obtain an image with sufficient quality to allow for a reasonable interpretation of the FAF findings (see Chap. 4, Fig. 4.4).

In essence, abnormal FAF signals either derive from a change in the number or composition of fluorophores in the RPE cell cytoplasm (i.e., lipofuscin) or from the presence of absorbing or autofluorescent material anterior to the RPE monolayer (Figs. 8.2 and 8.3). In addition, abnormal tissue with fluorophores with spectral characteristics similar to RPE-lipofuscin at the level of the choroid may cause a corresponding increased FAF signal (Fig. 8.4).

As outlined in the previous chapters and demonstrated in the clinical part of this book, it must be noted that FAF imaging provides information over and above conventional imaging techniques. Therefore, the identification of a pathological change on funduscopy such as drusen under the RPE may not give a clue as to the associated autofluorescence characteristics of these changes. For example, the FAF signal may be normal, decreased, or increased, depending on the molecular composition of the drusen material (more or fewer fluorophores) and the corresponding alteration of the overlying RPE (more or less flattening and reduction in lipofuscin granule density; see Chap. 11). While drusen in association with monogenetic juvenile macular dystrophies tend to be associated with an increased FAF signal, this is usually not the case for drusen in the context of complex, multifactorial age-related macular degeneration.

For the evaluation and interpretation of a FAF image in a individual patient, it may be helpful to correlate the findings with those obtained with reflectance images of the same excitation wavelength and other imaging methods, including fundus photographs, optical coherence tomography, and fluorescein angiography.

Below are the major causes and pathophysiologic categories for increased or reduced FAF signals.

Causes for a reduced FAF signal:

Reduction in RPE lipofuscin density
- RPE atrophy (such as geographic atrophy)
- Hereditary retinal dystrophies (such as RPE65 mutations)

Increased RPE melanin content
- e.g., RPE hypertrophy

Absorption from extracellular material/cells/fluid anterior to the RPE
- Intraretinal fluid (such as macular edema)
- Migrated melanin-containing cells
- Crystalline drusen or other crystal-like deposits
- Fresh intraretinal and subretinal hemorrhages

- Fibrosis, scar tissue, borders of laser scars
- Retinal vessels
- Luteal pigment (lutein and zeaxanthin)
- Media opacities (vitreous, lens, anterior chamber, cornea)

Causes for an increased FAF signal:

Excessive RPE lipofuscin accumulation
- Lipofuscinopathies, including Stargardt disease, Best disease, pattern dystrophy, and adult vitelliform macular dystrophy
- Age-related macular degeneration, such as RPE in the junctional zone preceding enlargement of occurrence of geographic atrophy

Occurrence of fluorophores anterior or posterior to the RPE cell monolayer
- Intraretinal fluid (such as macular edema)
- Subpigment epithelial fluid in pigment epithelial detachments
- Drusen in the subpigment epithelial space
- Migrated RPE cells or macrophages containing lipofuscin or melanolipofuscin (seen as pigment clumping or hyperpigmentation on funduscopy)
- Older intraretinal and subretinal hemorrhages
- Choroidal vessel in the presence of RPE and choriocapillaris atrophy, such as in the center of laser scars or within patches of RPE atrophy
- Choroidal nevi and melanoma

Lack of absorbing material
- Depletion of luteal pigment, such as in idiopathic macular telangiectasia type 2
- Displacement of luteal pigment, such as in cystoid macular edema

Optic nerve head drusen

Artefacts

Acknowledgements

The authors thank Adnan Tufail and Andrew R. Webster at Moorfields Eye Hospital for their help in the collection of images.

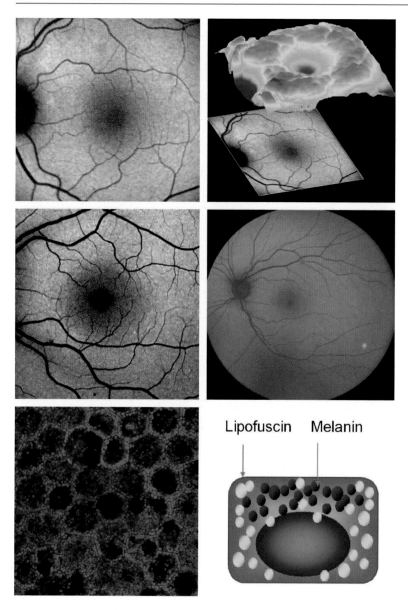

Fig. 8.1 *Top row:* Normal fundus autofluorescence (FAF) images obtained with a confocal scanning laser ophthalmoscope (Heidelberg Retina Angiograph). The FAF image shows the spatial distribution of the intensity of the FAF signal for each pixel in gray values. By definition, low pixel values (dark) illustrate low intensities, and high pixel values *(bright)* illustrate high intensities. In the normal subject, dark-appearing retinal vessels due to absorption from blood contents, a dark optic nerve head due to absence of autofluorescent material, and an increased signal in the macular area secondary to absorption from luteal pigment (lutein and zeaxanthin) can be observed. The relative distribution of FAF intensities can also be illustrated in pseudo-three-dimensional reconstruction techniques *(right)*. Areas with low FAF intensities are shown in *blue* and can be distinguished from the normal background signal *(red)*. *Middle row:* Modern imaging systems allow visualization of more details (in the presence of clear media and optimal patient cooperation) and the ability to image even larger retinal areas with up to a 55° field. Note the interindividual differences in macula pigment absorption between these examples from normal subjects.

Fig. 8.1 *(Continued) Bottom row:* Confocal scanning laser microscope image of the polygonal retinal pigment epithelium cell monolayer *(left)* and schematic drawing *(right)* showing a predominant location of lipofuscin granules *(red)* at the peripheral cell margin, while absorbing melanin granules are oriented toward the apical cell center and the cell nucleus at the basal side

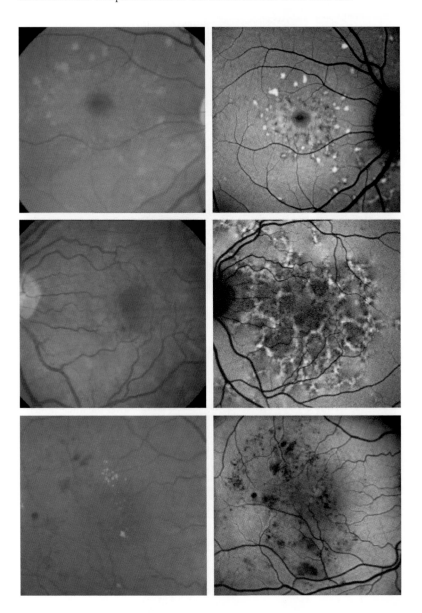

Fig. 8.2 *Top row:* Example of increased fundus autofluorescence (FAF) signals *(right)* corresponding to funduscopically visible *(left)* yellowish lesions in a patient with Stargardt disease. *Middle row:* Example of increased FAF signal corresponding to funduscopically visible yellowish and in part hyperpigmented, reticular lesions in a patient with pattern dystrophy. *Bottom row:* Example of increased FAF image signal corresponding to macular edema in the presence of diabetic maculopathy. Exudates and hemorrhages are characterized by low FAF levels due to absorption phenomena. Additional areas with decreased intensity can be observed and appear to be normal on fundus photography

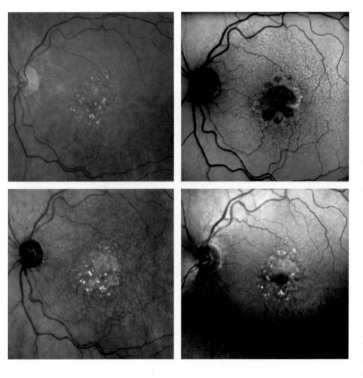

Fig. 8.3 Example of decreased fundus autofluorescence (FAF) corresponding to retinal pigment epithelium atrophy and crystalline drusen in a patient with geographic atrophy secondary to age-related macular degeneration. Levels of increased FAF can be observed surrounding the atrophy as retinal areas with excessive lipofuscin accumulation. For comparison, near-infrared reflectance (*lower left*) and blue-light reflectance (*lower right*) are illustrated as well. Note also prominent reticular drusen outside atropic patches (see chapter 11.4)

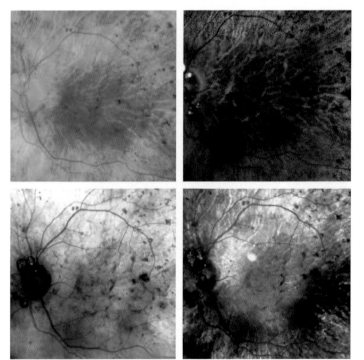

Fig. 8.4 Example of marked ey decreased fundus autofluorescence (FAF) intensity over the whole posterior pole in the presence of severe retinal pigment epithelium (RPE) atrophy in a patient with Usher syndrome. Underlying choroidal vessels that are usually obscured by the RPE can now be observed on FAF imaging by levels of increased FAF. Note that optic disc drusen are present, showing increased FAF. For comparison, near-infrared reflectance (*lower left*) and blue-light reflectance (*lower right*) are illustrated as well

Part II
Clinical Application

Macular and Retinal Dystrophies

9

Andrea von Rückmann, Fredrick W. Fitzke,
Steffen Schmitz-Valckenberg, Andrew R. Webster, Alan C. Bird

It is well established that autofluorescent material accumulates in the retinal pigment epithelium (RPE) in many macular and retinal dystrophies and that the extracellular deposits may also fluoresce. However, until recently information has been limited because observations have been made as a result of histological studies alone. It is unknown whether variance in fundus autofluorescence (FAF) is consistent from one condition to another, and the time course of the accumulation of autofluorescent material has not been documented. Given that many disorders are involved that are presumed to have different underlying defects, some variation might be expected from one condition to another. It is evident that in-vivo recording of RPE autofluorescence would allow many more observations to be made and that recording lipofuscin accumulation may give important clues as to the pathogenesis and progress of a number of retinal diseases.

Various alterations of the normal distribution of FAF intensities have been described in macular and retinal dystrophies. Funduscopically visible pale yellowish deposits at the level of the RPE/Bruch's membrane in Best disease, adult vitelliform macular dystrophy, and Stargardt macular dystrophy/fundus flavimaculatus are spatially confined to markedly increased FAF intensities [4, 25]. Focal flecks in Stargardt disease are much more clearly delineated on FAF images compared with fundus photographs. They show a bright FAF signal that may fade as atrophy develops. These findings are in accordance with histopathological data that have shown that these flecks represent aggregates of enlarged RPE cells engorged to 10 times their normal size with lipofuscin [6, 13, 24]. In a clinical study, including electrophysiological tests, of 43 patients with Stargardt disease, Lois and coworkers demonstrated a functional correlate of FAF abnormalities [9, 10]. They showed that low levels of FAF intensity in the fovea were associated with peripheral cone and rod dysfunction, whereas no functional abnormalities in patients with normal or high FAF signal could be measured (see Chap. 10). As in all forms of macular dystrophies examined systematically to date, background autofluorescence in Stargardt disease appears to be elevated, implying a generalised abnormality of the RPE [25]. This observation confirms the impression derived from histological studies that inherited macular dystrophies affect the entire RPE.

Using FAF imaging, there is no correlation with the fluorescein angiographic sign of a dark choroid. Lorenz and colleagues described absent or minimal FAF intensities in patients with early-onset severe retinal dystrophy associated with mutations on both allels of RPE65 (see Fig. 9.9) [11]. The lack or severe decrease of FAF signal would be consistent with the biochemical defect and could be used as a clinical marker of this genotype. Another study demonstrated that patients with Leber's congenital amaurosis having vision reduced to light perception and undetectable electroretinograms may still exhibit normal or minimally decreased FAF intensities [22]. This suggests that the RPE/photoreceptor complex is, at least in part, functionally and anatomically intact. This finding would have implications for future treatment, indicating that photoreceptor function may still be rescuable in such patients.

In patients with vitelliform macular dystrophies, FAF patterns have been described as spokelike, diffuse, or a combination of the two [2, 23]. It has been speculated that these areas with increased FAF do not represent lipofuscin accumulation at the level of the RPE but rather shed photoreceptor outer segments associated with sub-retinal fluid.

FAF imaging may show abnormal distributions of intensities in subjects with mutations known to cause macular and retinal dystrophy but with no manifest ophthalmoscopic or functional abnormalities. This means that this technique allows detection of the abnormal phenotype in some disorders when it is not otherwise evident. In Figs. 9.1–9.18, FAF findings in different macular and retinal dystrophy are illustrated.

References

1. Bellmann, C, Neveu, MM, Scholl, HP, et al. (2004) Localized retinal electrophysiological and fundus autofluorescence imaging abnormalities in maternal inherited diabetes and deafness. Invest Ophthalmol Vis Sci 45:2355–2360

2. Chung, JE, Spaide, RF (2004) Fundus autofluorescence and vitelliform macular dystrophy. Arch Ophthalmol 122:1078–1079

3. Cideciyan, AV, Swider, M, Aleman, TS, et al. (2005) ABCA4-associated retinal degenerations spare structure and function of the human parapapillary retina. Invest Ophthalmol Vis Sci 46:4739–4746

4. Delori, FC, Dorey, CK, Staurenghi, G, et al. (1995) In vivo fluorescence of the ocular fundus exhibits retinal pigment epithelium lipofuscin characteristics. Invest Ophthalmol Vis Sci 36:718–729

5. Downes, SM, Payne, AM, Kelsell, RE, et al. (2001) Autosomal dominant cone–rod dystrophy with mutations in the guanylate cyclase 2D gene encoding retinal guanylate cyclase-1. Arch Ophthalmol 119:1667–1673

6. Eagle, RC, Jr., Lucier, AC, Bernardino, VB, Jr., Yanoff, M (1980) Retinal pigment epithelial abnormalities in fundus flavimaculatus: a light and electron microscopic study. Ophthalmology 87:1189–1200

7. Jarc-Vidmar, M, Kraut, A, Hawlina, M (2003) Fundus autofluorescence imaging in Best's vitelliform dystrophy. Klin Monatsbl Augenheilkd 220:861–867

8. Jarc-Vidmar, M, Popovic, P, Hawlina, M (2006) Mapping of central visual function by microperimetry and autofluorescence in patients with Best's vitelliform dystrophy. Eye 20:688–696

9. Lois, N, Holder, GE, Bunce, C, et al. (2001) Phenotypic subtypes of Stargardt macular dystrophy-fundus flavimaculatus. Arch Ophthalmol 119:359–369

10. Lois, N, Halfyard, AS, Bird, AC, et al. (2004) Fundus autofluorescence in Stargardt macular dystrophy-fundus flavimaculatus. Am J Ophthalmol 138:55–63

11. Lorenz, B, Wabbels, B, Wegscheider, E, et al. (2004) Lack of fundus autofluorescence to 488 nanometers from childhood on in patients with early-onset severe retinal dystrophy associated with mutations in RPE65. Ophthalmology 111:1585–1594

12. Massin, P, Guillausseau, PJ, Vialettes, B, et al. (1995) Macular pattern dystrophy associated with a mutation of mitochondrial DNA. Am J Ophthalmol 120:247–248

13. McDonnell, PJ, Kivlin, JD, Maumenee, IH, Green, WR (1986) Fundus flavimaculatus without maculopathy. A clinicopathologic study. Ophthalmology 93:116–119

14. Michaelides, M, Johnson, S, Tekriwal, AK, et al. (2003) An early-onset autosomal dominant macular dystrophy (MCDR3) resembling North Carolina macular dystrophy maps to chromosome 5. Invest Ophthalmol Vis Sci 44:2178–2183

15. Miller, SA (1978) Fluorescence in Best's vitelliform dystrophy, lipofuscin, and fundus flavimaculatus. Br J Ophthalmol 62:256–260

16. Nakazawa, M, Wada, Y, Tamai, M (1995) Macular dystrophy associated with monogenic Arg172Trp mutation of the peripherin/RDS gene in a Japanese family. Retina 15:518–523

17. Nichols, BE, Sheffield, VC, Vandenburgh, K, et al. (1993) Butterfly-shaped pigment dystrophy of the fovea caused by a point mutation in codon 167 of the RDS gene. Nat Genet 3:202–207

18. O'Gorman, S, Flaherty, WA, Fishman, GA, Berson, EL (1988) Histopathologic findings in Best's vitelliform macular dystrophy. Arch Ophthalmol 106:1261–1268

19. Renner, AB, Tillack, H, Kraus, H, et al. (2004) [Clinical diagnostic prerequisites for adult vitelliform macular dystrophy]. Ophthalmologe 101:895–900

20. Renner, AB, Tillack, H, Kraus, H, et al. (2004) Morphology and functional characteristics in adult vitelliform macular dystrophy. Retina 24:929–939

21. Robson, AG, Egan, CA, Luong, VA, et al. (2004) Comparison of fundus autofluorescence with photopic and scotopic fine-matrix mapping in patients with retinitis pigmentosa and normal visual acuity. Invest Ophthalmol Vis Sci 45:4119–4125

22. Scholl, HP, Chong, NH, Robson, AG, et al. (2004) Fundus autofluorescence in patients with leber congenital amaurosis. Invest Ophthalmol Vis Sci 45:2747–2752

23. Spaide, RF, Noble, K, Morgan, A, Freund, KB (2006) Vitelliform macular dystrophy. Ophthalmology 113:1392–1400

24. Steinmetz, RL, Garner, A, Maguire, JI, Bird, AC (1991) Histopathology of incipient fundus flavimaculatus. Ophthalmology 98:953–956

25. von Rückmann, A, Fitzke, FW, Bird, AC (1997) In vivo fundus autofluorescence in macular dystrophies. Arch Ophthalmol 115:609–615

26. von Rückmann, A, Schmidt, KG, Fitzke, FW, et al. (1998) [Fundus autofluorescence in patients with hereditary macular dystrophies, malattia leventinese, familial dominant and aged-related drusen]. Klin Monatsbl Augenheilkd 213:81–86

27. Wabbels, B, Preising, MN, Kretschmann, U, et al. (2006) Genotype-phenotype correlation and longitudinal course in ten families with Best vitelliform macular dystrophy. Graefes Arch Clin Exp Ophthalmol 244:1453–1466

28. Wabbels, B, Demmler, A, Paunescu, K, et al. (2006) Fundus autofluorescence in children and teenagers with hereditary retinal diseases. Graefes Arch Clin Exp Ophthalmol 244:36–45

Fig. 9.1 Stargardt macular dystrophy/fundus flavimaculatus, early stage. Fundus photographs and fundus autofluorescence (FAF) images (30° and montage) of a 27-year-old woman with 6/60 visual acuities in both eyes. In early stages, FAF imaging typically shows a central oval area of reduced signal surrounded by small disseminated spots of reduced and increased intensity [10, 28]. Central retinal pigment epithelium (RPE) atrophy is also present, showing very decreased FAF intensity. At the periphery, fundus photographs show well-defined yellowish deposit at the level of the RPE. These flecks correspond to punctate spots with bright FAF signal. They can be better delineated and their number appear to be greater on the FAF images. The montage images demonstrate that the spots with markedly increased signal are scattered over the whole fundus

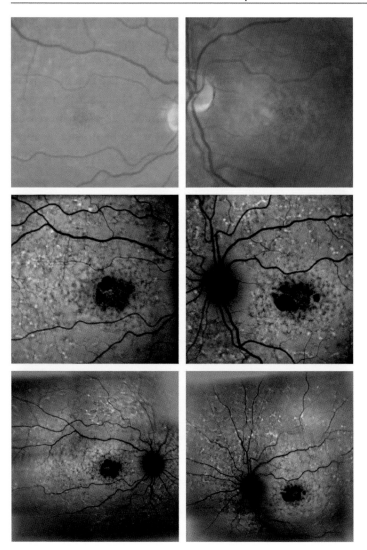

Fig. 9.2 Stargardt macular dystrophy/fundus flavimaculatus, late stage. Fundus photographs and fundus autofluorescence (FAF) montage of a 48-year-old man diagnosed with Stargardt disease more than 20 years previously. There is extensive multi-focal retinal pigment epithelium atrophy in the macula, showing levels of severe decreased FAF signal. The retinal periphery shows marked alteration of normal background signal with disseminated areas of increased and decreased intensity. Note that the FAF signal appears to be normal around the optic nerve head (peripapillary sparing), a typical finding in patients with Stargardt disease (see also Fig. 9.1) [3]

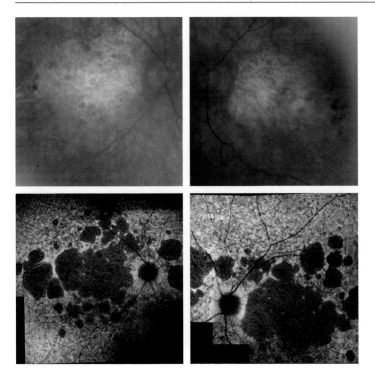

Fig. 9.3 Best vitelliform macular dystrophy. *Top row:* Reflectance and fundus autofluorescence (FAF) image of the left eye of a 10-year-old boy (vitelliform stage). A well-defined white deposit centrally at the level of the retinal pigment epithelium (RPE) is observed. Visual acuity with the left eye was 6/6. FAF imaging shows an increased signal that corresponds with the deposit but also extends outside the lesion as seen on ophthalmoscopy [7, 8, 15, 18, 25, 27]. The surrounding fundus is relatively more fluorescent than age-matched normal subjects. *Middle row:* FAF images of both eyes in a 21-year-old man. Visual acuities were 6/6 for the right and 6/5 for the left. The right eye (vitelliruptive stage) shows levels of increased FAF inside the central lesion, particularly at the bottom. In the very center, decreased intensity can be observed, indicating incipient RPE atrophy. FAF imaging of the left eye discloses a level of increased FAF at the borders of the lesion with a very bright signal at the bottom (pseudo-hypopyon stage). *Bottom row:* Fundus photograph and FAF image of the left eye of a 65-year-old woman (atrophic stage). Visual acuity with the left eye was 6/9. Previous electrophysiology had shown a normal electroretinogram but a pathological electro-oculogram with no light rise. The central area of RPE atrophy exhibits a much decreased FAF signal. Note that that there is a second lesion in the superior macula in the vitelliruptive stage showing a mottled increased FAF signal

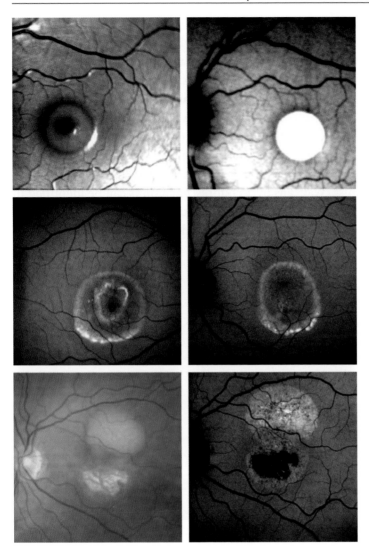

Fig. 9.4 Adult-onset vitelliform macular dystrophy. *Top and middle rows:* Fundus photograph, fundus autofluorescence (FAF) image, and early- and late-phase fluorescein angiogram of a 48-year-old man presenting with a gradual decrease in visual function over the previous years. Electrophysiology disclosed a borderline electro-oculogram but no typical findings for Best disease. There is whitish-yellow deposit at the central macula, which corresponds to marked increased autofluorescence [2, 19, 20, 23, 25]. Early angiography shows hypofluorescence due to masking effects. A late-phase angiogram disclosed hyperfluorescence with staining of the lesion. Furthermore, basal laminar deposits ("stars in the sky," "Milky Way") as hyperfluorescence spots can be identified in the outer macula. *Bottom row:* Reflectance and FAF image 12 months later. The central lesion has undergone disruption with mottled spots of marked increased FAF signal

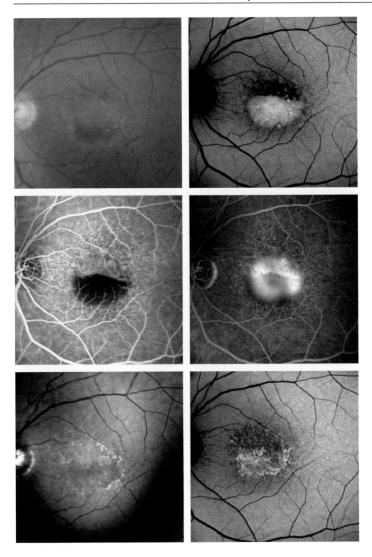

Fig. 9.5 Adult-onset vitelliform macular dystrophy. *Top row:* Left eye of a 75-year-old woman with adult vitelliform macular dystrophy with a well-defined white deposit at the level of the retinal pigment epithelium centrally and visual acuity of 6/18. She had no family history, and her vision had been stable for years. Very marked enhanced autofluorescence signal corresponds with the deposit. *Middle row:* Fundus photograph and fundus autofluorescence (FAF) image of the right eye of a 76-year-old woman, visual acuity 1/60. Vision in the left eye had recently deteriorated. Electrophysiology disclosed an abnormal pattern electroretinogram but a normal Ganzfeld electroretinogram and a normal electro-oculogram. FAF imaging shows levels of increased and decreased intensity inside the central lesion, implying the beginning of retinal pigment epithelium (RPE) atrophy. *Bottom row:* Reflectance and FAF images of a 53-year-old man with adult vitelliform macular dystrophy and an atrophic lesion at the level of the RPE centrally. Right eye visual acuity was 6/60. Autofluorescence imaging showed decreased signal that corresponded to the atrophic area. The surrounding fundus was relatively more fluorescent than in age-matched normal subjects

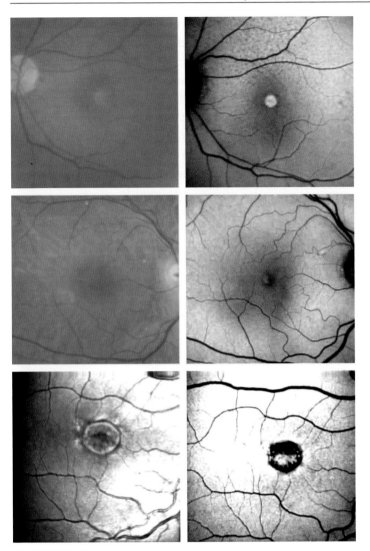

Fig. 9.6 Dominant drusen/Doyne honeycomb maculopathy/malattia leventinese. Fundus autofluorescence (FAF) images and fundus photographs in patients with dominant drusen [14]. Autofluorescence imaging typically reveals levels of increased intensity corresponding to funduscopically visible drusen areas [26]. This observation is in contrast to hard and small drusen in patients with age-related macular degeneration, which usually show normal or slightly decreased autofluorescence (see Chap. 11). *Top left:* Areas of marked decreased intensity in patients with dominant drusen may be caused by atrophy of the retinal pigment epithelium. *Bottom line:* This patient was tested positive for fibulin-3 gene mutation

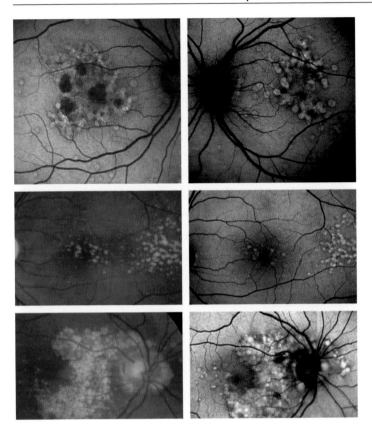

Fig. 9.7 Three examples of typical retinal manifestation in maternal inherited diabetes and deafness (MIDD) syndrome. *Top row:* Left eye of 48-year-old man; *middle and bottom rows:* right and left eyes of 52-year-old man. Genetic testing confirmed mitochondrial DNA nucleotide A3243G point mutation in both patients [1, 12]. Fundus photography shows irregular patches of paramacular atrophy, pale sub-retinal deposits, and pigment clumping with sparing of the foveal center. Using fundus autofluorescence imaging, pericentral circumferential atrophy is clearly visualized by decreased intensity. There is diffuse irregular autofluorescent adjacent to atrophy. Note that both the peripapillary region and the foveal center appear to exhibit normal background signal

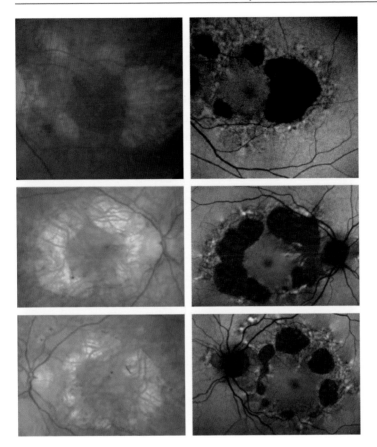

Fig. 9.8 Macular dystrophy. Fundus photographs and fundus autofluorescence (FAF) images of a 50-year-old man. No prominent abnormalities can be observed on fundus photography, whereas FAF imaging shows severe alterations in the central macula with levels of decreased and increased intensities. Note the symmetrical pattern between the eyes. The FAF montage shows that the disease appears to be limited to the central macula, which is consistent with electrophysiological findings disclosing an abnormally pattern electroretinogram but a normal Ganzfeld electroretinogram

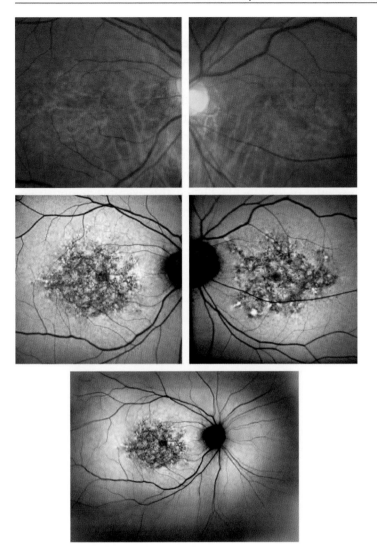

Fig. 9.9 Dominantly inherited pattern dystrophy. Fundus photographs and fundus autofluorescence (FAF) images of a mother (*first and second rows*) and son (*third and fourth rows*) from a family with known autosomal-dominant pattern dystrophy (mutation: RDS Arg172Trp) [16]. The mother had reduced vision for years. Autofluorescence imaging shows extensive changes with levels of increased and decreased intensity involving the entire macula. A parafoveal ring of increased intensity is also present. The 17-year-old son had no visual complaints (visual acuity 6/6 in both eyes). Although fundus photographs reveal no obvious abnormality, autofluorescent imaging shows an oval area of marked increased intensity in the center of the macula. Hence, this example demonstrates the abilities of FAF imaging to identify an abnormal phenotype when it is not otherwise evident

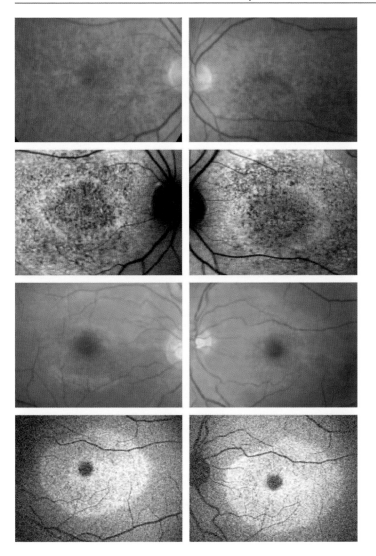

Fig. 9.10 Dominantly inherited pattern dystrophy. *Top and middle rows:* Near-infrared reflectance and corresponding fundus autofluorescence (FAF) images of a 55-year-old woman with pattern dystrophy (mutation in the peripherin/ *RDS* gene) [17]. Autofluorescence imaging shows a bilateral butterfly-shaped area of increased intensity. There are also speckled areas of decreased signal inside the central lesion, indicating incipient atrophy. *Bottom row:* FAF images of a patient with pattern dystrophy presenting with a different phenotype. A macro-reticular pattern with areas of increased autofluorescence is observed. Small areas of parafoveal atrophy are characterised by markedly decreased intensity and can be clearly distinguished from decreased autofluorescence because of macula pigment absorption

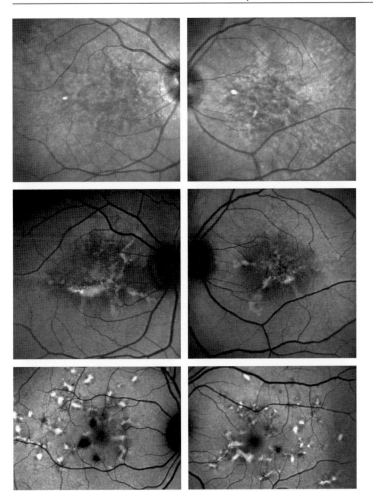

Fig. 9.11 Dominantly inherited macular dystrophy. *Top and middle rows:* Fundus photographs and fundus autofluorescence (FAF) images of a 23-year-old woman with no visual complaints. Visual acuities were 6/5 in both eyes. Fundus photographs show subtle central yellow deposits. The autofluorescence signal is markedly abnormal, exhibiting areas of increased intensity and therefore strongly suggestive of an abnormal phenotype. *Bottom row:* FAF images of the woman's mother (60 years old at presentation, visual acuity 6/36 in both eyes), showing central retinal pigment epithelium atrophy surrounded by areas of irregularly increased intensity. She had noticed visual problems at 46 years of age. Her own mother lost vision with age, implying a dominant inheritance pattern with affection in three generations

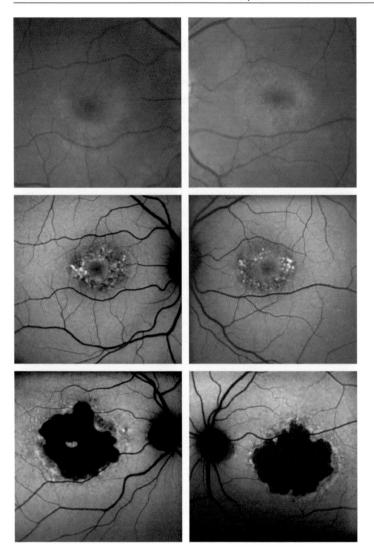

Fig. 9.12 Cone and cone-rod dystrophy (GCAP-1). Fundus autofluorescence (FAF) images of patients with mutations in the guanylate cyclase activator 1A gene encoding guanylate cyclase activating protein-1 [5]. *Top row:* A 41-year-old woman with abnormal generalised cone dysfunction on electrophysiology. FAF images show symmetrically bilateral bull's-eye-shaped lesions with decreased intensity and a surrounding ring of increased autofluorescence. This lesion was hardly visible on fundus photography. *Middle row:* Only subtle autofluorescence changes with loss of macula pigment absorption and marked increased autofluorescence are present in early stages. *Bottom row:* In later stages, areas of focally decreased intensity or—even later—of markedly decreased autofluorescence due to the development of atrophy are observed. Note that the ring of increased signal surrounding the lesion is visible in advanced stages as well

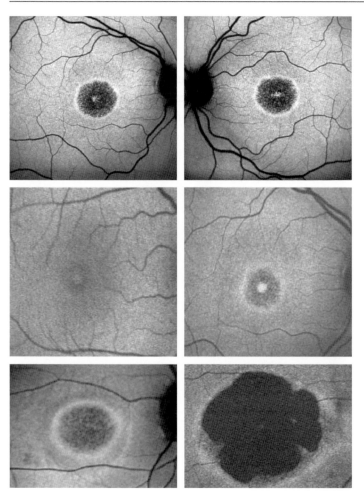

Fig. 9.13 Cone dystrophy. Fundus photographs and fundus autofluorescence (FAF) images of a 40-year-old man with visual acuities of 6/60 in the right eye and 1/60 in the left. He had noticed visual problems 4 years previously. Electro-diagnostic testing revealed generalized cone dysfunction and supernormal rod function. Fundus photography shows symmetrically bilateral foveal bull's-eye lesions. The FAF characteristics are unusual with mainly levels of increased intensity [5]. There are also small areas with decreased intensity inside the lesion, indicating development of retinal pigment epithelium atrophy. These areas with decreased signal are more prominent in the left eye, which corresponds with visual acuity measurement. One year later (*bottom row*), FAF imaging shows only subtle changes over time

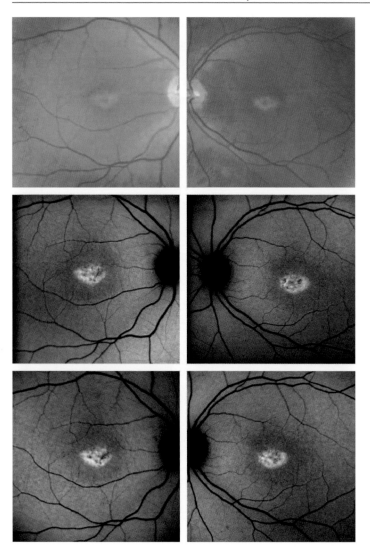

Fig. 9.14 Retinitis pigmentosa. Fundus photographs, fundus autofluorescence (FAF) images, and near-infrared reflectance images of a 22-year-old woman with retinitis pigmentosa 18. Visual acuities were 6/6 in the right eye and 6/18 in the left. Pattern and Ganzfeld electroretinograms were both abnormal, whereas rod exceeded cone dysfunction. There are no obvious macular changes on the fundus photograph or reflectance image. By contrast, FAF imaging shows a typical ring of increased intensity (see also Chap. 9)

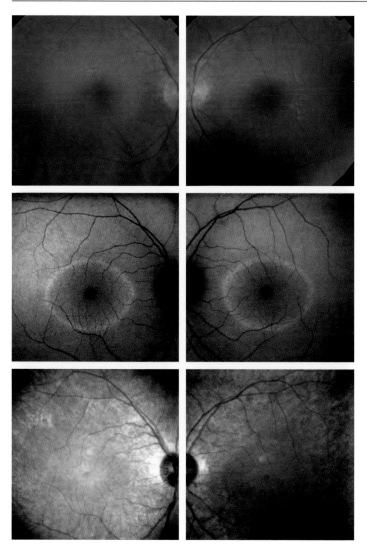

Fig. 9.15 Retinitis pigmentosa. *Top and middle rows:* Fundus autofluorescence (FAF) images of both eyes of a 51-year-old man with a presumably autosomal-recessive inheritance pattern. In addition to the ring of increased FAF, severe retinal pigment epithelium changes can be visualized in the peripheral retina with levels of increased and decreased autofluorescence [21]. *Bottom row:* Patient with sector retinitis pigmentosa. FAF imaging clearly shows the involved areas in the inferior retina. The ring of increased intensity appears to be interrupted at the superior macula

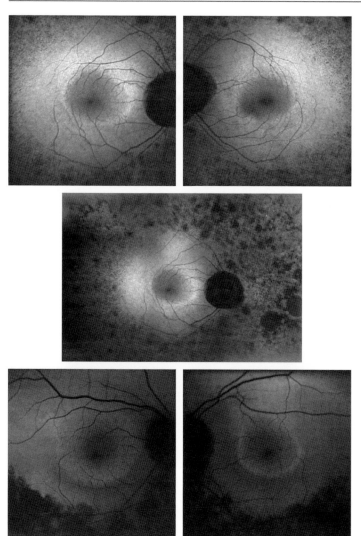

Fig. 9.16 Retinitis pigmentosa, Usher syndrome. Fundus photographs and fundus autofluorescence (FAF) images of two patients with Usher syndrome type 2. Central visual acuity was preserved. Visual field testing showed extensive constriction corresponding to the central area of normal-appearing FAF intensity. Note that the extension and presence of morphological abnormalities can be much better visualized with FAF imaging

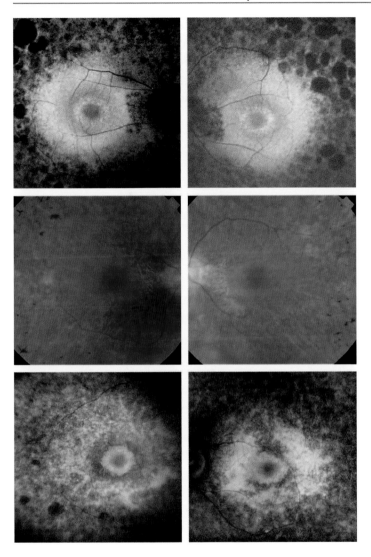

Fig. 9.17 Bietti crystalline corneoretinal dystrophy. Fundus photographs, fundus autofluorescence (FAF) image, blue-light reflectance image, and fluorescein angiogram of a 25-year-old woman. The autofluorescence background signal is severely reduced. Furthermore, reticular-like structures with increased intensity can be observed that do not seem to be related to any other structures seen on the other imaging modalities

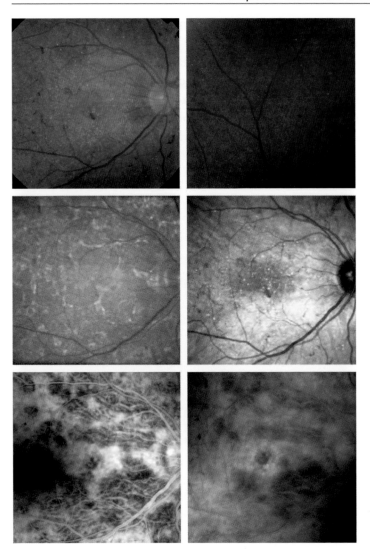

Fig. 9.18 X-linked retinoschisis. *Top row:* Fundus autofluorescence (FAF) images of a 35-year-old man with retinoschisis. FAF imaging showed levels of increased and decreased intensity in the central macula due to compression of the neural elements containing luteal pigment. Note part of an oval ring at the inferior retina of the right eye, corresponding to clinically visible retinoschisis. *Middle and bottom row:* Fundus photographs, horizontal OCT scans and FAF images of another patient with X-linked retinoschisis showing a similar FAF phenotype

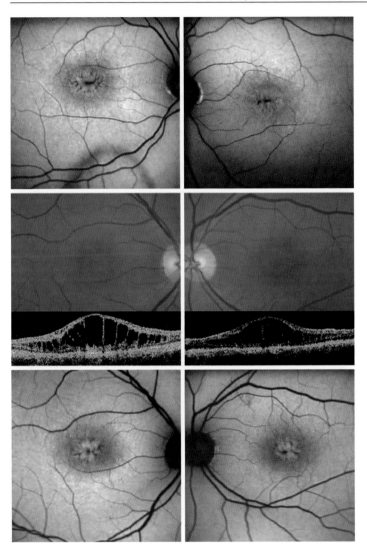

Fig. 9.19 Choroideremia. This 42 year old male with a long history of choroi-deremia had visual acuities of 6/6 in the right and 6/9 in the left eye. Fundus autofluorescence imaging *(middle row)* reveals a severely reduced background signal and visualizsation of underlying choroidal vessels. The preserved island in the central retina can be easily identified and corresponds to flourescein angiography findings *(bottom row)*. Note that the fundus photography *(top row)* and fluorescein angiography were performed two years before FAF imaging

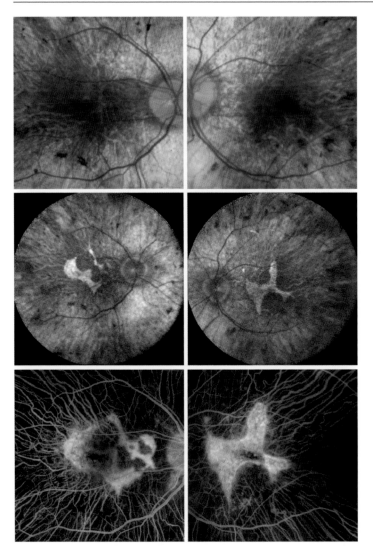

Discrete Lines of Increased Fundus Autofluorescence in Various Forms of Retinal Dystrophies

10

Monika Fleckenstein, Hendrik P.N. Scholl, Frank G. Holz

10.1
Introduction

Discrete, well-defined lines of increased fundus autofluorescence (FAF) may occur in various forms of retinal dystrophies [1–12]. These lines usually have no visible correlate on fundus biomicroscopy or fluorescein angiography and are thought to originate from excessive fluorophore (e.g. in lipofuscin granules) accumulation at the level of the retinal pigment epithelium (RPE) cell monolayer. There is evidence from combined functional investigations that these lines reflect the border of impaired retinal sensitivity [2–4, 8–10]. Despite the variable orientation of this line in different entities—such as orientation along the retinal veins in pigmented paravenous chorioretinal atrophy (PPCRA) or a ring structure in retinitis pigmentosa (RP) or cone-rod dystrophy (CRD)—the similar appearance on FAF images and the concordance of functional findings indicate that these lines in heterogeneous diseases entities share a common underlying pathophysiologic mechanism.

10.2
Different Orientation of Lines of Increased FAF

10.2.1
Orientation Along Retinal Veins

Orientation of such a line along retinal veins can be observed in patients diagnosed with PPCRA (Figs. 10.1a). The phenomenon of orientation of the progressive atrophy of deep retinal layers including the RPE and the choriocapillaris along anteriorly located larger retinal venous vessels is obscure. It may be speculated that the topographic distribution of the deep changes results from a release of cytokines from vascular cellular elements, and thus "communication" with anatomic levels beneath the inner retina may play a role. It is remarkable that the orientation of the line of increased

FAF along the retinal veins of eyes at more advanced stages of PPCRA (Fig. 10.1a, left eye) finally appears to result in the formation of a ring-like structure in the parafoveal region. This finding may also indicate a related pathomechanism leading to formation and constriction of the parafoveal ring in RP.

10.2.2
Ring Shape

A line of increased FAF in the form of a parafoveal ring of variable eccentricity has been described in patients with RP [1–4, 8–11] (Fig. 10.2a), Leber's congenital amaurosis (LCA) [5], CRD [6, 7, 9, 11], and X-linked retinoschisis (XLRS) [12].

A ring of increased FAF can be detected in some patients with RP and normal visual acuity and has been demonstrated to surround areas of normal FAF. In some patients, the ring has been shown to constrict progressively over time [10]. It is still unknown why such a ring is not found in all patients with RP who demonstrate clinical evidence of macular sparing. Two LCA patients exhibiting a ring of increased FAF have recently been described [5]. Despite severe visual impairment, the ring is surrounded by almost normal FAF. By contrast, in the reports on a ring of increased FAF in CRD [6, 7, 9, 11], and XLRS [12], respectively, the ring has been reported to encircle areas of reduced or absent FAF, corresponding to macular atrophy.

10.3
Functional Correlate of Lines/Rings of Increased FAF

Functional analyses of the line/ring of increased FAF have been performed in RP [3, 4, 8–10] and CRD [9].

In RP it has been demonstrated that patients with larger FAF rings also had larger central visual fields [3, 4, 8, 10]. Furthermore, Robson and colleagues first showed a high correlation between the pattern electroretinogram (ERG) P50 amplitude—a valuable indicator of macular function—and the size of the abnormal ring [3]. Using fine matrix mapping, they could further demonstrate that photopic sensitivity was preserved over central macular areas, but there was a gradient of sensitivity loss over high-density segments of the ring and severe threshold elevation outside the arc of the ring. Scotopic sensitivity losses were more severe, and they encroached on areas within the ring [4].

Popovic and co-workers confirmed by fundus perimetry that retinal sensitivity was preserved within the ring and was lost outside the ring regardless of whether the FAF pattern was normal or whether atrophic lesions of the RPE were already present or not [8]. (Fig. 10.2c shows the fundus perimetry in a patient with autosomal-dominant RP.)

It has been concluded that the ring of increased FAF in RP demarcates areas of preserved central photopic function and that constriction of the ring may mirror progressive visual field loss by advancing dysfunction that encroaches over areas of central macula [3, 4, 10].

There are few reports about rings of increased FAF in CRD [6, 7, 9]. In the majority of these patients, the ring encircles areas of central atrophy (Fig. 10.3a). Functional assessment has been performed in only a few patients with CRD [9]: Robson et al. could demonstrate that the pattern ERG P50 amplitude was inversely related to the size of the FAF ring; by fine-matrix mapping they revealed a gradient of sensitivity loss across the arc of increased FAF.

In a patient with macular dystrophy (Fig. 10.3), who displayed a ring of increased FAF that surrounded areas of decreased/absent FAF, fundus perimetry revealed (Figs. 10.3c) that within the ring, independent of a normal or abnormal FAF signal, there was light sensitivity loss. Outside the ring, the FAF signal and light sensitivity were almost normal. These findings were exactly opposite to the findings in RP where the central sensitivity was preserved (Fig. 10.2c).

Despite a different orientation of the line in PPCRA, fundus perimetry has revealed that the area with impaired sensitivity exceeded the area of RPE cell loss and was precisely delineated (Figs. 10.1c). In the central retina and in the periphery that was not framed by the line, the FAF signal was normal, and light sensitivity was preserved. Within the area outlined by increased FAF, independently of a normal or abnormal FAF signal, there was impaired light sensitivity. These observations are in accordance with the findings in RP whereby the ring or line of increased FAF represented the border between functional and dysfunctional light sensitivity.

At this interface, there may be a higher phagocytic and, thus, metabolic load of the corresponding RPE cells, with subsequent excessive accumulation of fluorophores in the lysosomal compartment resulting in a line of increased signal that can be visualized by FAF imaging. It is remarkable that the FAF signal on both sides of this demarcation line in most of these cases was normal or near normal (Figs. 10.1a, 10.2a, 10.3a), although on one side, there was impaired sensitivity.

Robson and colleagues suggested that restoration of normal FAF intensity over concentric areas outside the ring in RP may indicate continued but possibly impaired phagocytosis and removal of abnormal material, or that it could be explained by loss of photoreceptor cells [3, 4, 10]. Scholl et al. concluded that normal or near-normal FAF may be present in areas of photoreceptor dysfunction and that a normal FAF reflects the presence of structurally intact photoreceptors and the integrity of the photoreceptor/RPE complex rather than normal photoreceptor function [5].

In the few histopathological reports from eyes with RP, it has been noted that despite obvious photoreceptor degeneration, the RPE may display only minor morphological abnormalities. It was hypothesised that there is a high capacity of the "young" RPE to compensate for excessive photoreceptor cell degeneration before the RPE cell layer eventually suffers collateral damage and, finally, cell death [13].

It remains unknown whether such areas could be prevented from progressive cell death; they therefore represent potential targets for future therapies designed to restore vision at the photoreceptor level.

In summary, a line of increased FAF in various retinal dystrophies appears to represent the demarcation of impaired retinal sensitivity, independent of its orientation and the localisation of phatologic alterations. This phenomenon may therefore represent a non-specific finding in different disease entities and points to a common downstream pathogenetic pathway.

References

1. von Rückmann A, Fitzke FW, Bird AC, Autofluorescence imaging of the human fundus. In: Marmor MF, Wolfensberger TJ (eds) (1998) The retinal pigment epithelium. Oxford University Press, Oxford

2. Holder GE, Robson AG, Hogg CR, et al. (2003) Pattern ERG: clinical overview, and some observations on associated fundus autofluorescence imaging in inherited maculopathy. Doc Ophthalmol 106:17–23

3. Robson AG, El-Amir A, Bailey C, et al. (2003) Pattern ERG correlates of abnormal fundus autofluorescence in patients with retinitis pigmentosa and normal visual acuity. Invest Ophthalmol Vis Sci 44:3544–3550

4. Robson AG, Egan CA, Luong VA, et al. (2004) Comparison of fundus autofluorescence with photopic and scotopic fine-matrix mapping in patients with retinitis pigmentosa and normal visual acuity. Invest Ophthalmol Vis Sci 45:4119–4125

5. Scholl HP, Chong NH, Robson AG, et al. (2004) Fundus autofluorescence in patients with leber congenital amaurosis. Invest Ophthalmol Vis Sci 45:2747–2752

6. Ebenezer ND, Michaelides M, Jenkins SA, et al. (2005) Identification of novel RPGR ORF15 mutations in X-linked progressive cone–rod dystrophy (XLCORD) families. Invest Ophthalmol Vis Sci 46:1891–1898

7. Michaelides M, Holder GE, Hunt DM, et al. (2005) A detailed study of the phenotype of an autosomal dominant cone–rod dystrophy (CORD7) associated with mutation in the gene for RIM1. Br J Ophthalmol 89:198–206

8. Popovic P, Jarc-Vidmar M, Hawlina M (2005) Abnormal fundus autofluorescence in relation to retinal function in patients with retinitis pigmentosa. Graefes Arch Clin Exp Ophthalmol 243:1018–1027

9. Robson A, Michaelides M, Webster A, et al. (2005) Comparison of pattern ERG, multifocal ERG and psychophysical correlates of fundus autofluorescence abnormalities in patients with cone–rod (RPGR, RIM1) or rod–cone dystrophy [ARVO abstract]. Invest Ophthalmol Vis Sci 43:552

10. Robson AG, Saihan Z, Jenkins SAm et al. (2006) Functional characterisation and serial imaging of abnormal fundus autofluorescence in patients with retinitis pigmentosa and normal visual acuity. Br J Ophthalmol 90:472–479

11. Wabbels B, Demmler A, Paunescu K, et al. (2006) Fundus autofluorescence in children and teenagers with hereditary retinal diseases. Graefes Arch Clin Exp Ophthalmol 244:36–45

12. Tsang SH, Vaclavik V, Bird AC, et al. (2007) Novel phenotypic and genotypic findings in X-linked retinoschisis. Arch Ophthalmol 125:259–267

13. Farber DB, Flannery JG, Bird AC, et al. (1987) Histopathological and biochemical studies on donor eyes affected with retinitis pigmentosa. Prog Clin Biol Res 247:53–67

Fig. 10.1 FAF image (**a**), fundus photograph (**b**), and fundus perimetry (shown with colour-coded scale) superimposed on the FAF image (**c**) in a patient with bilateral PPCRA. A line of increased FAF that is oriented along the retinal veins can be detected (**a**) that shows no prominent correlate in fundus photography (**b**). In the left eye, this line almost merges to a ring-like structure in the para-foveal region (**a**, *right side*). Fundus perimetry reveals that this line almost pre-cisely reflects the border of preserved light sensitivity; on both sides of this line, the FAF signal is normal/near normal; however, on one side there is severely impaired light sensitivity (**c**)

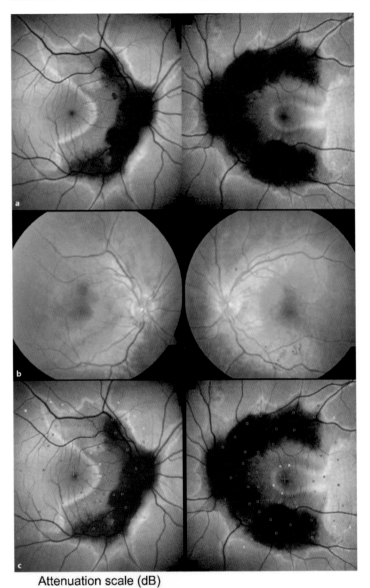

Attenuation scale (dB)

0 2 4 6 8 10 12 14 16 18 20

Fig. 10.2 FAF image (**a**), fundus photograph (**b**), and fundus perimetry (shown with colour-coded scale) superimposed on FAF image (**c**) in a patient with bilateral autosomal-dominant retinitis pigmentosa. The ring of increased FAF surrounds an area displaying a normal FAF signal (**a**). Fundus perimetry reveals normal light sensitivity within the ring. Despite a normal FAF signal outside this ring, there is severely impaired light sensitivity (**c**)

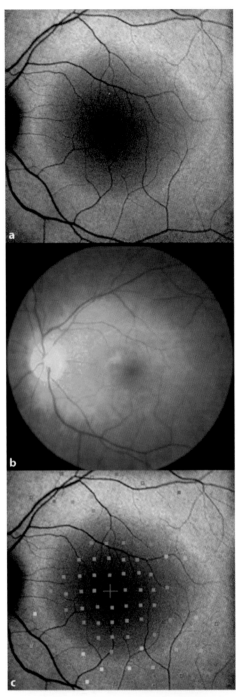

Attenuation scale (dB)

0 2 4 6 8 10 12 14 16 18 20

Fig. 10.3 FAF image (**a**), fundus photograph (**b**), and fundus perimetry (shown with colour-coded scale) superimposed on FAF image (**c**) in a patient diagnosed with bilateral macular dystrophy. The ring of increased FAF encircles an area that clearly shows reduced FAF centrally and a normal FAF signal between the centre and the ring of increased FAF (**a**). Within the ring, there is severely impaired light sensitivity independent of the normal or reduced FAF signal; outside the ring, sensitivity is almost normal (**c**)

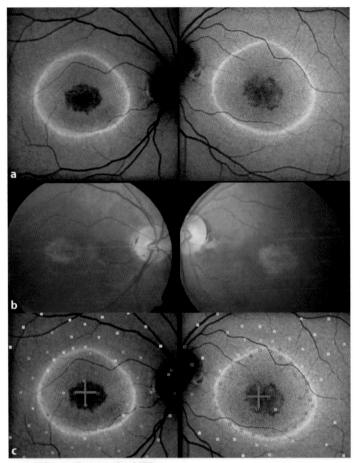

Attenuation scale (dB)

0 2 4 6 8 10 12 14 16 18 20

Age-Related Macular Degeneration I — Early Manifestation

11

Steffen Schmitz-Valckenberg, Hans-Martin Helb,
Almut Bindewald-Wittich, Samantha S. Dandekar, Frank G. Holz

11.1
Background

Age-related macular degeneration (AMD), a complex disease with both genetic and environmental factors, has become the most common cause of legal blindness in industrialised countries [4, 7–9, 12, 17]. The pathophysiologic mechanisms underlying the disease process are still incompletely understood, but a key role in the disease process has been attributed to the retinal pigment epithelium (RPE).

A hallmark of ageing is the accumulation of lipofuscin (LF) granules in the cytoplasm of RPE cells. Several lines of evidence indicate that adverse effects of excessive LF accumulation represent common downstream pathogenetic mechanisms in various blinding hereditary and complex retinal diseases, including AMD. Furthermore, recent experimental data suggest links between accumulation of LF and inflammation, complement system activation, and oxidative damage [19].

Fundus autofluorescence (FAF) imaging as a modality to map metabolic changes of RPE LF accumulation in vivo has been studied recently in patients with AMD. These analyses include the spatial correlation of FAF findings with established early AMD changes such as focal hypo- and hyperpigmentation and drusen.

11.2
FAF Findings

One important observation in patients with early AMD is that alterations in the FAF signal are not necessarily associated with corresponding funduscopically or angiographically visible changes such as drusen and irregular hyper- or hypopigmentations (Figs. 11.1–11.3) [2, 3, 10, 16, 18]. This indicates that FAF findings may represent an independent measure of disease stage and activity.

In comparisons with the normal background signal, it has been demonstrated that corresponding drusen areas can exhibit levels of increased, decreased, or normal autofluorescence intensities. In the latter case, drusen are invisible on FAF images. Some patients with very early AMD may even have no FAF changes at all, showing the normal homogenous background FAF over the whole posterior pole (Fig. 11.1, top row). The absence of any FAF abnormalities in the presence of soft or hard drusen could be caused by masking effects of yellow macular pigment or by the image resolution and quality if individual drusen are small (<60 μm). Larger drusen are associated more frequently with more pronounced FAF abnormalities than smaller ones are. When several small hard or soft drusen convalesce, multiple foci and/or irregular areas of FAF can be observed (Fig. 11.1, middle and bottom rows). Crystalline drusen are characterised by a decreased FAF signal secondary to absorption phenomena. Several authors have consistently reported that confluent drusen and large foveal soft drusen (drusenoid RPE detachments) topographically correspond well with patchy, mildly increased FAF (Fig. 11.2, top row) [3, 10, 13]. It has been speculated that such FAF alteration may represent a reduced turnover and a net increase in the amount of LF. Interestingly, longitudinal observations by Einbock et al. suggest that this patchy pattern correlates with a particularly high risk for the development of choroidal neovascularizations [6].

Another interesting finding in patients with early AMD is the observation of FAF variations in the vicinity of drusen (Fig. 11.2, middle and bottom rows). Focal areas of increased FAF in the neighbourhood of drusen may occur, commonly in areas with pigment clumping or adjacent to long-standing and mineralised drusen areas [18]. These focal changes next to drusen may also be spatially confined to focal hyperpigmentation at the level of the RPE and correspond to dark areas on fluorescein angiography. Increased FAF intensities over focal hyperpigmentation and pigment figures have been explained by the presence of melanolipofuscin or changes in the metabolic activity of the RPE [14, 18]. Areas of hypopigmentation on fundus photographs tend to be associated with a corresponding decreased FAF signal, suggesting the absence of RPE cells or degenerated RPE cells with a reduced content of fluorophores and/or LF granules.

Delori and colleagues have described a pattern of FAF distribution associated with drusen that consists of decreased FAF in the center of the druse and surrounded, in most cases, by an annulus of increased FAF [5]. Decreased FAF intensities over the center of the druse are probably not caused by melanin pigment and are not as low as areas of RPE atrophy. These observations would be more consistent with a peripheral displacement of the overlying RPE cytoplasm over the drusen, causing central thinning of RPE and a peripheral increase in intensities and/or LF granules, rather than with manifest RPE atrophy.

Recent approaches to investigate FAF findings in AMD patients include the use of image analysis software to topographically map FAF alterations to fundus photographs or reflectance images and to compare pixel values [13, 15]. New findings with these approaches include significant differences in focal increased FAF intensities between eyes of various AMD manifestations. Using the fundus camera of FAF imaging, Spaide reported that eyes with early AMD manifestation of patients with exudative AMD in the fellow eye had larger amounts of areas with abnormal autofluorescence than did eyes with early AMD manifestation in patients witout a history of exudative AMD in the fellow eye. In contrast, Smith et al. reported in another analysis that fellow eyes of patients with unilateral exudative AMD tended not to exhibit FAF abnormalities obtained with the cSLO. The analysis of pixel values is limited by the image resolution, macula pigment distribution, non-standardised imaging protocols, and the relatively low reproducibility of subtle FAF alterations with regards to both localisation and magnitude. Furthermore, the comparison of findings that are obtained by different imaging systems (using different excitation and emission filters) and that are analysed by different image analysis protocols is challenging and may explain at least some of the inconsistencies in the results of different approaches.

11.3
Classification of FAF Patterns in Early AMD

An analysis of the variability of FAF findings in patients with early AMD was recently published by an international workshop on FAF phenotyping in early AMD [3]. Pooling data from several retinal centres, researchers developed a classification system with eight different FAF patterns (Figs. 11.1–11.3). This classification demonstrates the relatively poor correlation between visible alterations on fundus photography and notable FAF changes. Based on these results, it was speculated that FAF findings in early AMD may indicate more widespread abnormalities and diseased areas. The changes seen in FAF imaging on the RPE cell level may precede the occurrence of visible lesions as the disease progresses. It is still unknown whether phenotypic diagnosed AMD is pathophysiologically and genetically a uniform disease. Therefore, the introduced classification system may help in identifying specific high-risk characteristics for disease progression as well as in designing and monitoring future interventional trials. Furthermore, phenotyping based on FAF imaging may be used for molecular genetic analysis to identify one or several genes conferring risk for the development of certain AMD manifestations.

11.4
Reticular Drusen

Reticular drusen, or so-called reticular pseudodrusen, are a relatively common finding on FAF images in patients with AMD. While it remains unclear whether they represent a distinct risk factor for development of choroidal neovascularization (CNV), preliminary data suggest that reticular drusen are more prevalent in AMD patients compared with subjects in the same age group [1, 11]. Reticular drusen can be identified as a peculiar pattern on FAF images, with multiple relatively uniform roundish or elongated spots with decreased intensities and surrounded by an interlacing network of normal-appearing FAF signals (Fig. 11.4) [3]. They appear to be more pronounced and widespread superior and superior-temporal to the fovea, but extend towards the large temporal vascular arcade as well as nasally of the optic disc. In some patients, a similar pattern with deep yellowish-orange spots can be seen on fundus photographs or with a similar mosaic appearance on reflectance images or fluorescein angiography. Overall, reticular drusen are readily identified on FAF images and more easily detected than on funduscopy or fundus photographs. However, the particular nature of these alterations is not yet clearly understood, including the morphological substrate and the exact anatomic location (i.e. sub-RPE, Bruch's membrane, choriocapillaris).

References

1. Arnold, JJ, Sarks, SH, Killingsworth, MC, Sarks, JP (1995) Reticular pseudodrusen: a risk factor in age-related maculopathy. Retina 15:183–191

2. Bellmann, C, Holz, FG, Schapp, O, et al. (1997) [Topography of fundus autofluorescence with a new confocal scanning laser ophthalmoscope]. Ophthalmologe 94:385–391

3. Bindewald, A, Bird, AC, Dandekar, SS, et al. (2005) Classification of fundus autofluorescence patterns in early age-related macular disease. Invest Ophthalmol Vis Sci 46:3309–3314

4. Bird, A (1996) Age-related macular disease. Br J Ophthalmol 80:2–3

5. Delori, FC, Fleckner, MR, Goger, DG, et al. (2000) Autofluorescence distribution associated with drusen in age-related macular degeneration. Invest Ophthalmol Vis Sci 41:496–504

6. Einbock, W, Moessner, A, Schnurrbusch, UE, et al. (2005) Changes in fundus autofluorescence in patients with age-related maculopathy. Correlation to visual function: a prospective study. Graefes Arch Clin Exp Ophthalmol 243:300–305

7. Holz, FG, Pauleikhoff, D, Spaide, RF, Bird, AC (2004) Age-related macular degeneration. Springer, Berlin

8. Holz, FG, Pauleikhoff, D, Klein, R, Bird, AC (2004) Pathogenesis of lesions in late age-related macular disease. Am J Ophthalmol 137:504–510

9. Klein, R, Klein, BE, Tomany, SC, et al. (2002) Ten-year incidence and progression of age-related maculopathy: the Beaver Dam eye study. Ophthalmology 109:1767–1779

10. Lois, N, Owens, SL, Coco, R, et al. (2002) Fundus autofluorescence in patients with age-related macular degeneration and high risk of visual loss. Am J Ophthalmol 133:341–349

11. Maguire, MG, Fine, SL (1996) Reticular pseudodrusen. Retina 16:167–168

12. Mitchell, P, Smith, W, Attebo, K, Wang, JJ (1995) Prevalence of age-related maculopathy in Australia. The Blue Mountains Eye Study. Ophthalmology 102:1450–1460

13. Smith, RT, Chan, JK, Busuoic, M, et al. (2006) Autofluorescence characteristics of early, atrophic, and high-risk fellow eyes in age-related macular degeneration. Invest Ophthalmol Vis Sci 47:5495–5504

14. Solbach, U, Keilhauer, C, Knabben, H, Wolf, S (1997) Imaging of retinal autofluorescence in patients with age-related macular degeneration. Retina 17:385–389

15. Spaide, RF (2003) Fundus autofluorescence and age-related macular degeneration. Ophthalmology 110:392–399

16. Spital, G, Radermacher, M, Muller, C, et al. (1998) [Autofluorescence characteristics of lipofuscin components in different forms of late senile macular degeneration]. Klin Monatsbl Augenheilkd 213:23–31

17. van Leeuwen, R, Klaver, CC, Vingerling, JR, et al. (2003) Epidemiology of age-related maculopathy: a review. Eur J Epidemiol 18:845–854

18. von Rückmann, A, Fitzke, FW, Bird, AC (1997) Fundus autofluorescence in age-related macular disease imaged with a laser scanning ophthalmoscope. Invest Ophthalmol Vis Sci 38:478–486

19. Zhou, J, Jang, YP, Kim, SR, Sparrow, JR (2006) Complement activation by photooxidation products of A2E, a lipofuscin constituent of the retinal pigment epithelium. Proc Natl Acad Sci USA 103:16182–16187

Fig. 11.1 Classification of fundus autofluorescence (FAF) patterns in early age-related macular degeneration with fundus photograph (*left*) and FAF image (*right*)—part 1. Normal (*top row*): homogenous background FAF and a gradual decrease in the inner macula towards the fovea due to the masking effect of macular pigment. Only small hard drusen are visible in the corresponding fundus photograph. Minimal change (*middle row*): only minimal variations from normal background FAF. There is limited irregular increase or decrease in FAF intensity due to multiple small hard drusen. Focal (*bottom row*): several well-defined spots with markedly increased FAF. Fundus photograph of the same eye with multiple hard and soft drusen

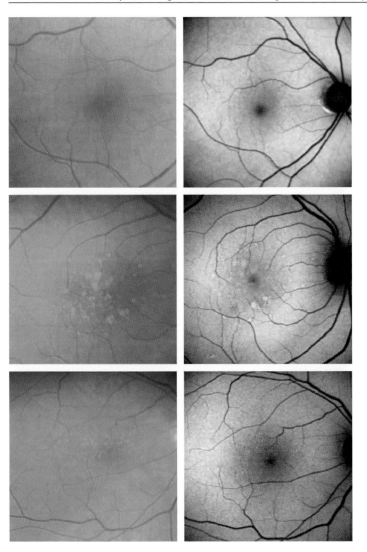

Fig. 11.2 Classification of fundus autofluorescence (FAF) patterns in early age-related macular degeneration with fundus photograph (*left*) and FAF image (*right*)—part 2. Patchy (*top row*): multiple large areas (>200 µm in diameter) of increased FAF corresponding to large, soft drusen and/or hyperpigmentation on the fundus photograph. Linear (*middle row*): characterised by the presence of at least one linear area with markedly increased FAF. A corresponding hyperpigmented line is visible in the fundus photograph. Lace-like (*bottom row*): multiple branching linear structures of increased FAF. This pattern may correspond to hyperpigmentation on the fundus photograph or there may be no visible abnormalities

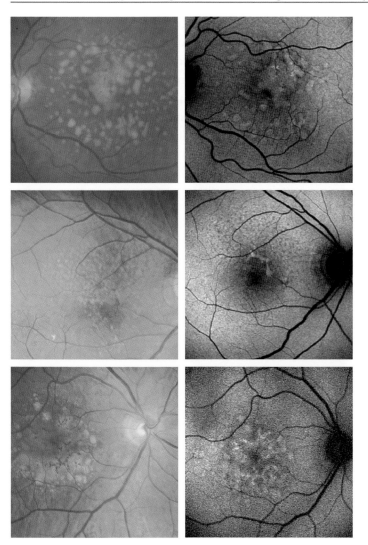

Fig. 11.3 Classification of fundus autofluorescence (FAF) patterns in early age-related macular degeneration with fundus photograph (*left*) and FAF image (*right*)—part 3. Reticular (*top row*): multiple, specific small areas of decreased FAF with brighter lines in between. The reticular pattern not only occurs in the macular area but is found more typically in a superotemporal location. There may be visible reticular drusen in the corresponding fundus photograph. Speckled (*bottom row*): a variety of FAF abnormalities in a larger area of the FAF image. There seem to be fewer pathologic areas in the corresponding fundus

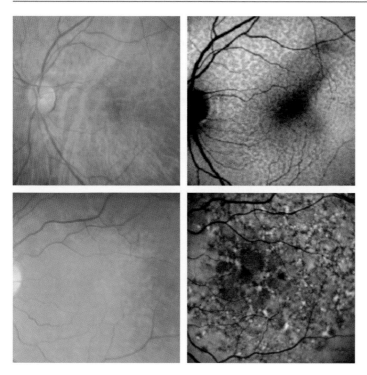

Fig. 11.4 Illustration of findings with various imaging methods for the left eye in a patient with juxtafoveal occult choroidal neovascularisation and reticular drusen. Reticular drusen can be clearly seen on the fundus autofluorescence (FAF) image (*top right*) by decreased intensities and surrounded by an interlacing network of normal-appearing FAF signal. A similar pattern can be suspected on the fundus photograph (*top left*). Corresponding spots can be seen on late-phase fluorescein angiography by hyperfluorescent spots (*middle right*) and on the late-phase indocyanine green (ICG) angiography by hypofluorescent spots (*bottom right*). Early-phase fluorescein (*left middle*) and early-phase ICG (*bottom left*) angiograms show only subtle changes

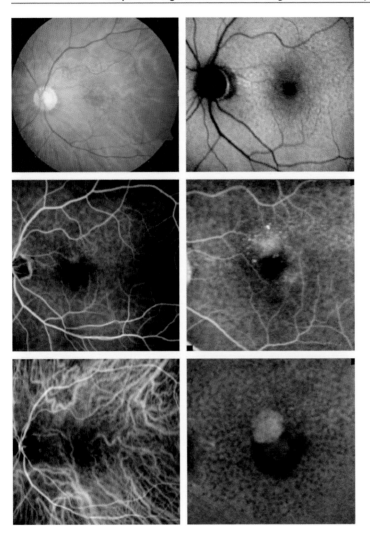

Age-Related Macular Degeneration II— Geographic Atrophy

12

Steffen Schmitz-Valckenberg, Almut Bindewald-Wittich,
Monika Fleckenstein, Hendrik P.N. Scholl, Frank G. Holz

12.1
Background

Geographic atrophy (GA) represents the atrophic late-stage manifestation of "dry" age-related macular degeneration (AMD). It is characterised by the development of atrophic patches that may initially occur in the parafoveal area [3, 13, 16, 23]. During the natural course of the disease, atrophy slowly enlarges over time, and the fovea itself is typically not involved until later ("foveal sparing", see Fig 12.3).

The pathophysiologic mechanisms underlying the disease process are not completely understood. It is thought that the accumulation of lipofuscin in the retinal pigment epithelium (RPE) cells is a by-product of incompletely digested photoreceptor outer segments and plays a key role in the disease process (see Chap. 1). Histopathologic studies have shown that clinically visible areas of atrophy are confined to areas with cell death of the RPE and collateral tissue layers, i.e. the choriocapillaris and the outer neurosensory retina [7, 14, 15]. Another important finding is the observation of lipofuscin and melanolipofuscin-filled RPE cells in the junctional zone between the atrophic and the normal retina, while areas of atrophy itself are characterised by a loss of RPE and, therefore, lipofuscin granules.

Fundus autofluorescence (FAF) findings in patients with GA secondary to AMD are in accordance with these in-vitro analyses (Fig. 12.1) [10, 27]. Due to the distinct changes of the topographic distribution of RPE lipofuscin, which is the dominant fluorophore for FAF imaging (see Chap. 2), the signal is markedly reduced over atrophic areas, while high-intensity FAF levels can be observed in the junctional zone surrounding the atrophic patches. These morphological changes are usually without any correlate on fundus photography or fluorescein angiography.

12.2
Detection and Quantification of Atrophy

Because of a marked reduction in FAF signal intensity, areas of atrophy can be readily visualized on FAF images. Borders to non-affected retinal areas can be accurately outlined with high image contrast, whereby the delineation is more accurate when compared with fundus photography (Fig. 12.1). In contrast to fluorescein angiography, FAF imaging represents a non-invasive imaging method and is less time-consuming. However, retinal areas with decreased FAF intensity can also represent drusen areas or—if present in the fovea—may be caused by macula pigment absorption. Very rarely, severe vitreous opacities can markedly block the excitation light and obscure the details of underlying atrophic areas (see Chap. 4, Fig. 4.3). However, these artefacts can usually be easily identified by reflectance images, and atrophic areas can be accurately detected [19]. Reflectance images are helpful to analyse areas with decreased FAF in the fovea in order to distinguish between macula pigment absorption and atrophic areas. For differentiation between large drusen and small areas of atrophy, it should be noted that even drusen can exhibit a decreased FAF signal, the intensity over areas of atrophy is typically even more reduced. These observations have been confirmed by systematic measurements using fundus spectrophotometry [5].

The advantages of FAF imaging in GA have been used to detect and precisely quantify atrophic areas on FAF images using customised image analysis software (Fig. 12.2) [4, 17]. This software allows the automated segmentation of atrophic areas by a region algorithm. Interfering retinal blood vessels that have a similar FAF intensity compared with atrophic areas are recognised by the software and can be excluded from the measurements. Further developments include the alignment of FAF images at different examinations using retinal landmarks in order to correct for different scan angles and magnifications. This allows accurate assessment of atrophy progression over time and can be used in longitudinal observations, including interventional trials.

12.3
Correlation of FAF Findings with Functional Impairment

In accordance with the histopathologic studies reporting that GA is not limited to the RPE but also involves the outer neurosensory retina, atrophic areas are associated with an absolute or relative severe scotoma [24, 25]. Furthermore, patients typically complain about decreased vision in dim illumination and decreased contrast sensitivity. Measurement of visual acuity does not correlate well with the total size of atrophy in earlier stages of the disease (Fig. 12.3). In the presence of parafoveal atrophy but sparing of the fovea itself, the patient may only be able to read single letters on a chart. Reading or recognising faces may not be possible because the residual island of normal functioning foveal retina is too small. Using advanced technology, more accurate testing of patients' visual abilities can be achieved, and functional impairment can be spatially correlated to morphological alterations, including changes seen on FAF imaging.

This is of particular interest for retinal areas surrounding atrophy, i.e. the junctional zone of atrophy. Combining FAF imaging with fundus perimetry, it has been shown that retinal sensitivity in this area is significantly reduced over areas with increased FAF intensities compared to areas with normal background signal [18]. Using fine-matrix mapping, it has been demonstrated that rod function is more severely affected than cone function over areas with increased FAF in patients with AMD [20]. These findings demonstrate a functional correlate of decreased retinal sensitivity and areas with increased FAF. This would be in accordance with experimental data showing that compounds of lipofuscin such as A2-E possess toxic properties and may interfere with normal RPE cell function (see Chap. 1). Because normal photoreceptor function is dependent on normal RPE function, in particular with regards to the constant phagocytosis of shed distal outer-segment stacks for photoreceptor cell renewal, a negative feedback mechanism could be proposed whereby cells with lipofuscin-loaded secondary lysosomes would phagocytose less shed photoreceptor outer segments, subsequently leading to impaired retinal sensitivity in areas with increased FAF intensity.

12.4
Classification of FAF Patterns in Geographic Atrophy

While the presence of atrophy represents a non-specific end-stage manifestation in various retinal degenerations, the identification of elevated levels of FAF intensities in the junctional zone of atrophy is of particular interest as these changes precede cell death and, therefore, absolute scotoma [9]. Of note, these areas with high FAF signal surrounding atrophy can usually not be identified by funduscopy or any other imaging method.

Early studies using FAF imaging have already reported interindividual differences in the distribution and appearance of these areas, while there was a high degree of intraindividual symmetry [1, 10]. Based on these observations, a systematic review within the FAM (Fundus Autofluorescence in Age-Related Macular Degeneration) study has been published, introducing a classification of FAF patterns in the junctional zone of atrophy in patient with GA secondary to AMD (Fig. 12.4) [2]. This classification was originally based only on morphological FAF alterations. It consists of five different patterns, while the diffuse pattern is divided into another five subtypes.

12.5
FAF Patterns and Progression Over Time

Natural history studies on patients with advanced atrophic AMD have demonstrated that there is a high variability among patients of atrophy progression over time [11, 22, 23]. Current data on the spread of atrophy suggest that there is a linear growth of atrophy over time and that the best predictor is the growth rate in the previous year (Fig. 12.2) [6]. Atrophy enlargement for very small atrophic areas (less than one disc area or about 2.5 mm²) has been shown to be less rapid compared with areas with larger total size of baseline atrophy; however, the overall great difference in atrophy progression between eyes (about 0–13.8 mm²/per year) could not be explained either by baseline atrophy or by any other tested demographic factor (Fig. 12.3) [26].

Longitudinal observations using FAF imaging in GA have reported that new atrophic patches and the spread of pre-existing atrophy solely occur in areas with abnormally high levels of FAF at baseline [9]. A more recent study with a limited data set of eight eyes stated that new atrophy would not specifically develop where areas of increased FAF had previously been observed [12].

Larger samples and longer review periods of up to 10 years permit further investigation of atrophy progression over time and do correlate it to other factors, including baseline atrophy and FAF findings. It has been shown that the extension of the total area with increased FAF surrounding atrophy at baseline in eyes has a strong positive correlation with atrophy progression rate over time (Fig. 12.3) [19]. Recently, two large natural-history studies have confirmed that baseline atrophy is not a major risk factor for atrophy enlargement [11, 22]. The analysis in the context of the FAM study with 195 eyes could demonstrate that the great variability and range in atrophy enlargement among patients could be largely explained by FAF abnormalities outside the atrophic patches. Application of the previous introduced classification system for FAF patterns in the junctional zone of atrophy showed that variable growth rates were significantly dependent on the specific phenotype at baseline. Eyes with the banded (median 1.81 mm²/year) and the diffuse (1.77 mm²/year) FAF patterns showed a more rapid atrophy enlargement compared with eyes without FAF abnormalities (0.38 mm²/year) and with the focal FAF pattern (0.81 mm²/year) (Figs. 12.5 and 12.6). Within the group with the diffuse pattern, eyes with a diffuse trickling pattern could be identified that exhibited an even higher spread rate (median 3.02 mm²/year) compared with the other diffuse types (1.67 mm²/year). Overall, phenotypic features of FAF abnormalities had a much stronger impact on atrophy progression than any other risk factor that has been addressed in previous studies of progression of GA due to AMD. The differences in atrophy enlargement among FAF phenotypes may reflect heterogeneity on the cellular and molecular levels in the disease process. Because there is a high degree of intraindividual symmetry, genetic determinants rather than non-specific ageing changes may be involved. Recent findings on the role of polymorphisms in the genes coding for complement factor H (CFH), factor B (BF), and LOC387715 are in accordance with the assumption that genetic factors may play a major role in the pathophysiology of AMD [8, 21].

Furthermore, these findings are consistent with the functional analysis in the junctional zone of atrophy (see section 12.3) and underscore the pathophysiologic importance of excessive lipofuscin accumulation in the context of GA. Overall, FAF imaging can be regarded as an important method (1) to investigate genotype/phenotype correlation in order to determine specific genetic factors in a complex, multifactorial disease such as AMD, and (2) to identify prognostic markers and high-risk characteristics for further atrophy progression. The latter may be particularly important not only for natural-history studies but also for interventional trials to test novel therapeutic approaches to halt or slow down the progression of GA.

References

1. Bellmann, C, Jorzik, J, Spital, G, et al. (2002) Symmetry of bilateral lesions in geographic atrophy in patients with age-related macular degeneration. Arch Ophthalmol 120:579–584

2. Bindewald, A, Schmitz-Valckenberg, S, Jorzik, J, et al. (2005) Classification of abnormal fundus autofluorescence patterns in the junctional zone of geographic atrophy in patients with age related macular degeneration. Br J Ophthalmol 89:874–878

3. Blair, CJ (1975) Geographic atrophy of the retinal pigment epithelium. A manifestation of senile macular degeneration. Arch Ophthalmol 93:19–25

4. Deckert, A, Schmitz-Valckenberg, S, Jorzik, J, et al. (2005) Automated analysis of digital fundus autofluorescence images of geographic atrophy in advanced age-related macular degeneration using confocal scanning laser ophthalmoscopy (cSLO). BMC Ophthalmol 5:8

5. Delori, FC, Fleckner, MR, Goger, DG, et al. (2000) Autofluorescence distribution associated with drusen in age-related macular degeneration. Invest Ophthalmol Vis Sci 41:496–504

6. Dreyhaupt, J, Mansmann, U, Pritsch, M, et al. (2005) Modelling the natural history of geographic atrophy in patients with age-related macular degeneration. Ophthalmic Epidemiol 12:353–362

7. Green, WR, Engel, C (1992) Age-related macular degeneration: histopathologic studies: the 1992 Lorenz E. Zimmermann Lecture. Ophthalmology 100:1519–1535

8. Haddad, S, Chen, CA, Santangelo, SL, Seddon, JM (2006) The genetics of age-related macular degeneration: a review of progress to date. Surv Ophthalmol 51:316–363

9. Holz, FG, Bellman, C, Staudt, S, et al. (2001) Fundus autofluorescence and development of geographic atrophy in age-related macular degeneration. Invest Ophthalmol Vis Sci 42:1051–1056

10. Holz, FG, Bellmann, C, Margaritidis, M, et al. (1999) Patterns of increased in vivo fundus autofluorescence in the junctional zone of geographic atrophy of the retinal pigment epithelium associated with age-related macular degeneration. Graefes Arch Clin Exp Ophthalmol 237:145–152

11. Holz, FG, Bindewald-Wittich, A, Fleckenstein, M, et al. (2007) Progression of geographic atrophy and impact of fundus autofluorescence patterns in age-related macular degeneration. Am J Ophthalmol 143:463–472

12. Hwang, JC, Chan, JW, Chang, S, Smith, RT (2006) Predictive value of fundus autofluorescence for development of geographic atrophy in age-related macular degeneration. Invest Ophthalmol Vis Sci 47:2655–2661

13. Maguire, P, Vine, AK (1986) Geographic atrophy of the retinal pigment epithelium. Am J Ophthalmol 102:621–625

14. Sarks, JP, Sarks, SH, Killingsworth, MC (1988) Evolution of geographic atrophy of the retinal pigment epithelium. Eye 2 (Pt 5):552–577

15. Sarks, SH (1976) Ageing and degeneration in the macular region: a clinico-pathological study. Br J Ophthalmol 60:324–341

16. Schatz, H, McDonald, HR (1989) Atrophic macular degeneration. Rate of spread of geographic atrophy and visual loss. Ophthalmology 96:1541–1551

17. Schmitz-Valckenberg, S, Jorzik, J, Unnebrink, K, Holz, FG (2002) Analysis of digital scanning laser ophthalmoscopy fundus autofluorescence images of geographic atrophy in advanced age-related macular degeneration. Graefes Arch Clin Exp Ophthalmol 240:73–78

18. Schmitz-Valckenberg, S, Bultmann, S, Dreyhaupt, J, et al. (2004) Fundus autofluorescence and fundus perimetry in the junctional zone of geographic atrophy in patients with age-related macular degeneration. Invest Ophthalmol Vis Sci 45:4470–4476

19. Schmitz-Valckenberg, S, Bindewald-Wittich, A, Dolar-Szczasny, J, et al. (2006) Correlation between the area of increased autofluorescence surrounding geographic atrophy and disease progression in patients with AMD. Invest Ophthalmol Vis Sci 47:2648–2654

20. Scholl, HP, Bellmann, C, Dandekar, SS, et al. (2004) Photopic and scotopic fine matrix mapping of retinal areas of increased fundus autofluorescence in patients with age-related maculopathy. Invest Ophthalmol Vis Sci 45:574–583

21. Scholl, HPN, Bindewald-Wittich, A, Schmitz-Valckenberg, S, et al. (2006) Correlation of CFH Y402h allele distribution and risk of progression of geographic atrophy in patients with age-related macular degeneration (AMD). Invest Ophthalmol Vis Sci 47:438[Arvo abstract]

22. Sunness, J, Margalit, E, Srikurnaran, D, et al. (2007) The long-term natural history of geographic atrophy from age-related macular degeneration. Ophthalmology 114:271–277

23. Sunness, JS (1999) The natural history of geographic atrophy, the advanced atrophic form of age-related macular degeneration. Mol Vis 5:25

24. Sunness, JS, Bressler, NM, Maguire, MG (1995) Scanning laser ophthalmoscopic analysis of the pattern of visual loss in age-related geographic atrophy of the macula. Am J Ophthalmol 119:143–151

25. Sunness, JS, Applegate, CA, Haselwood, D, Rubin, GS (1996) Fixation patterns and reading rates in eyes with central scotomas from advanced atrophic age-related macular degeneration and Stargardt disease. Ophthalmology 103:1458–1466

26. Sunness, JS, Gonzalez-Baron, J, Applegate, CA, et al. (1999) Enlargement of atrophy and visual acuity loss in the geographic atrophy form of age-related macular degeneration. Ophthalmology 106:1768–1779

27. von Ruckmann, A, Fitzke, FW, Bird, AC (1995) Distribution of fundus autofluorescence with a scanning laser ophthalmoscope. Br J Ophthalmol 79:407–412

Fig. 12.1 Fundus autofluorescence (FAF) imaging gives additional information above and beyond conventional imaging methods. Geographic atrophy appears as sharply demarcated areas with depigmentation and enhanced visualization of deep choroidal vessels on fundus photography (*top*) Atrophic patches can be clearly delineated by decreased intensity using FAF imaging (*middle*). Note that there are decreased FAF intensities in the foveal area (*middle right*) that are caused by absorption of macula pigment and not atrophy. In the junctional zone of atrophy, levels of marked FAF intensity can be observed that are not visible on fluorescein angiography or fundus photography (*bottom*). These distinct changes surrounding atrophy can also be visualized by a three-dimensional plot illustrating the topographic distribution of FAF intensities in false colour

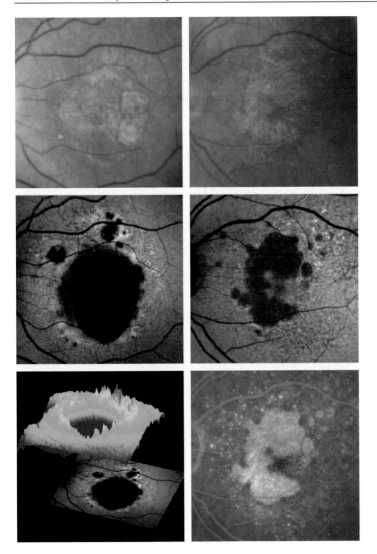

Fig. 12.2 *Top row:* Using image analysis software with customised, automated algorithms, interfering retinal vessels are identified, and atrophic areas are detected and quantified [4]. *Middle row:* Illustration of different image orientation between examinations due to different eye positions and laser scanning camera settings during fundus autofluorescence (FAF) acquisition by subtraction of baseline image from follow-up image. There is no useful overlay using the unprocessed images (*upper row*). In contrast, following the alignment of images using retinal blood vessels as landmarks, the spatial progression of atrophy over time can be clearly visualized (*lower row*). *Bottom row:* After alignment of images, the spread of atrophy and areas of increased FAF can be accurately analysed over time on FAF images (review period 3.5 years)

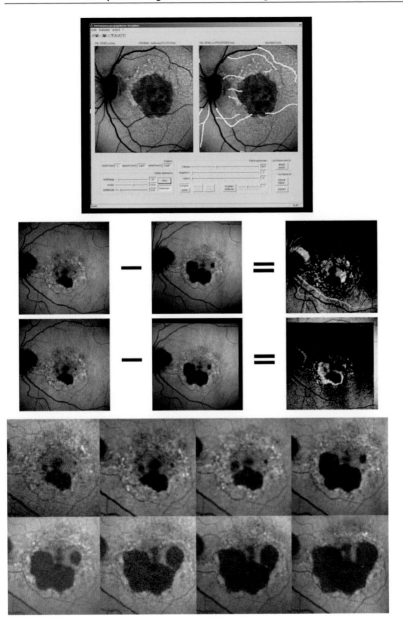

Fig. 12.3 *Top row:* Fundus autofluorescence (FAF) image and near-infrared reflectance image of the left eye of a patient with geographic atrophy secondary to age-related macular degeneration. There is extensive parafoveal atrophy with foveal sparing. Visual acuity was 6/9 in the left eye (fellow eye 6/60). However, the patient reported a marked increase in reading difficulties 2 months before presentation. FAF imaging indicates that the residual foveal island is obviously too small for reading words or text, while in routine clinical examination good central visual acuity is achieved. *Middle and bottom rows:* Illustration of the influence of baseline atrophy and FAF changes on atrophy progression over time. Although both eyes have similar sizes of baseline atrophy (*left column*), there is a great difference in the size of atrophy at the follow-up examination (review period for both examples about 6 years; *right column*), suggesting that baseline atrophy does not represent a major risk factor for atrophy progression. However, the area with increased FAF at baseline (delineated by the *polygon [convex hull]*) was much larger for the eye that showed a more rapid spread of atrophy

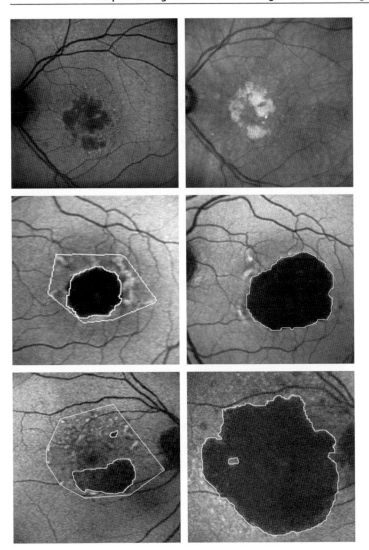

Fig. 12.4 Classification of fundus autofluorescence (FAF) patterns in the junctional zone in patients with geographic atrophy (GA) due to age-related macular degeneration. Eyes with no increased FAF intensity at all are graded as "none." The eyes with increased FAF are divided into two groups depending on the configuration of increased FAF surrounding the atrophy. Eyes showing areas with increased FAF directly adjacent to the margin of the atrophic patch(es) and elsewhere are called diffuse and are subdivided in five groups: *top row, left to right:* fine granular, branching; *bottom row, left to right:* trickling, reticular. and fine granular with punctuated spots. Eyes with increased FAF only at the margin of GA are split into three sub-types: focal, banded, and patchy, according to their typical FAF pattern around atrophy

Fig. 12.5 Illustration of the relationship between specific fundus autofluorescence (FAF) phenotypes and atrophy progression for patients with geographic atrophy due to age-related macular degeneration (part I—slow progressors) showing the baseline FAF image *(left)* and follow-up FAF image *(right)* for each eye, respectively. Eyes with no abnormal FAF changes (*top row,* atrophy progression 0.02 mm²/year, follow-up 12 months) and with only small areas of focally increased autofluorescence at the margin of the atrophic patch (*bottom row,* 0.36 mm²/year, follow-up 15 months) usually have a very slow progression over time

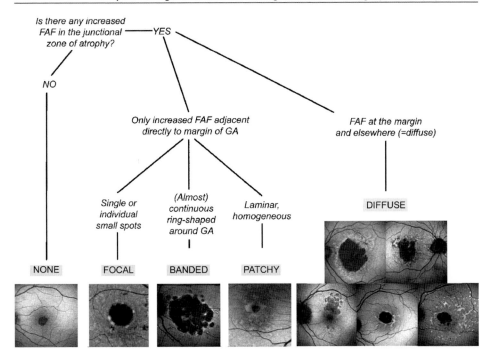

Is there any increased FAF in the junctional zone of atrophy? — YES

NO

Only increased FAF adjacent directly to margin of GA

FAF at the margin and elsewhere (=diffuse)

Single or individual small spots

(Almost) continuous ring-shaped around GA

Laminar, homogeneous

DIFFUSE

NONE

FOCAL

BANDED

PATCHY

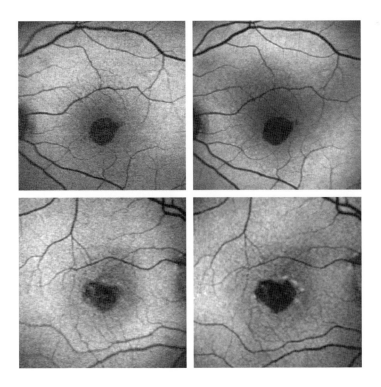

Fig. 12.6 Illustration of the relationship between specific fundus autofluorescence (FAF) phenotypes and atrophy progression for patients with geographic atrophy due to age-related macular degeneration (part II—rapid progressors) showing the baseline FAF image *(left)* and follow-up FAF image *(right)* for each eye, respectively. Eyes with the diffuse FAF pattern *(top row*, 1.71 mm²/year, follow-up 12 months) and with the banded type *(middle row*, 2.52 mm²/year, follow-up 18 months) of increased FAF surrounding atrophy are characterised by rapid atrophy enlargement. Very rapid atrophy progression can be observed in eyes with the diffuse trickling FAF pattern *(bottom*, 3.78 mm²/year, follow-up 18 months)

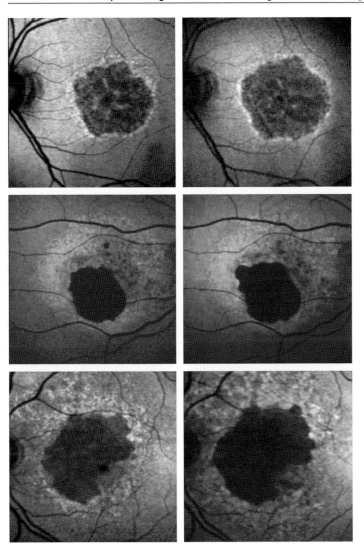

Felix Roth, Frank G. Holz

13.1
Introduction

Retinal pigment epithelial detachments (PEDs) are a common feature of advanced age-related macular degeneration (AMD; Figs. 13.1a, 13.2a, 13.3a). The accumulation of fluid between Bruch's membrane and the retinal pigment epithelial (RPE) cell monolayer is often associated with the accumulation of sub-neurosensory and intra-retinal oedema (Figs. 13.2b, 13.3b).

Over time, PEDs tend to enlarge gradually both in horizontal and vertical dimensions, and then flatten with the formation of subsequent subretinal fibrosis or atrophy associated with irreversible loss of neurosensory retinal function. The natural course also encompasses the development of a RPE tear, which may be associated with acute haemorrhages and additional visual loss (see Chap. 14.5) [3, 4, 6].

Detachments of the RPE from Bruch's membrane usually occur in association with occult choroidal neovascularization spreading under the RPE cell basal membrane or by retinal angiomatous proliferation (RAP). Based on angiographic findings, so-called serous PEDs may also develop in the absence of a neovascular membrane net. Given the constant fluid movements from the photoreceptor/RPE cell complex to the choroid, it has been speculated that barrier effects within Bruch's membrane may contribute by deposition of lipoidal constituents to the formation of such detachments. In particular, the accumulation of neutral lipids (cholesterol esters, triglycerides, diglycerides, and free fatty acids) would form a hydrophobic barrier that would impair the passage of fluid and result in accumulation of fluid in the sub-pigment epithelial space. RPE detachments would further be promoted by the mere presence of such deposits by decreasing adhesive forces between the RPE and Bruch's membrane [1–4, 6].

13.2
FAF Findings

Fundus autofluorescence (FAF) imaging in eyes with PED secondary to AMD, idiopathic central serous chorioretinopathy, or polypoidal choroidal vasculopathy shows variable FAF phenomena [5, 7–9]. Distinct variations of the normal background FAF signal in the area of the PED can be visualised, which are not detectable using conventional imaging techniques such as fundus photography, fluorescein, or indocyanine green angiography.

Changes in FAF intensities in patients with PED secondary to AMD can be classified into four groups. The majority of PEDs show a corresponding evenly marked and distributed *increase* of the FAF signal over the lesion, surrounded by a well-defined less autofluorescent halo delineating the entire border of the lesion (Figs. 13.1c, 13.2c). It has been speculated that the ring of decreased FAF at the edge of the PED may reflect beginning organisation of the lesion or may originate from absorption effects of sub-neurosensory extracellular fluid. There are also PEDs with an *intermediate* (Fig. 13.3d) or a *decreased* FAF signal over the lesion (Fig. 13.5c), which may or may not correspond to areas of RPE atrophy or fibrovascular scaring. Rarely, a PED shows a *cartwheel pattern* with corresponding hyperpigmented radial lines and a diminished autofluorescence signal between those lines (Fig. 13.6c).

Of note, changes in the FAF signal in the presence of PEDs are not necessarily caused by alterations of RPE lipofuscin accumulation. Other dominant fluorophores with similar excitation and emission spectra inside the PED, such as extracellular fluid or degraded photoreceptors, may be present and contribute to typical patterns with abnormal FAF intensity. The molecular species in the sub-RPE space remain to be identified. Overall, different FAF phenotypes may reflect not only different stages in the evolution of a PED (Fig. 13.4) but also heterogeneity on a cellular and molecular level in the disease process, and may thus be relevant for future molecular genetic analyses. Future longitudinal investigations are necessary to assess whether different phenotypic patterns are of predictive significance.

Fig. 13.1a–c Colour, fluorescein angiogram, and corresponding fundus auto-fluorescence (FAF) image showing a detachment of the retinal pigment epithelium due to age-related macular degeneration with increased FAF signal over the lesion and a surrounding area of decreased autofluorescence. Note the notch indicating occult choroidal neovascularisation in the fluorescein angiogram

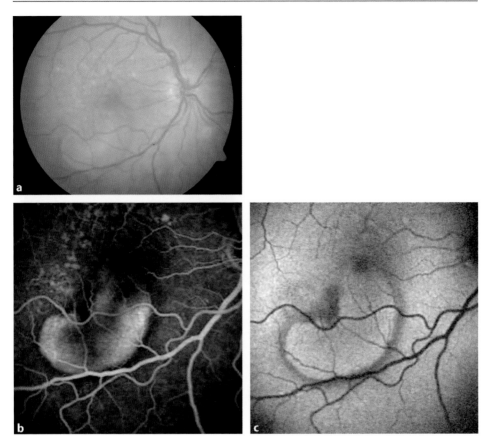

Fig. 13.2a–c Colour, optical coherence tomography, and corresponding fundus autofluorescence (FAF) image of a further detachment of the retinal pigment epithelium with increased FAF intensity over the lesion (possible RAP lesion)

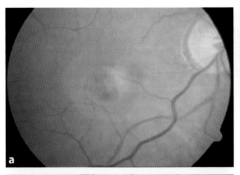

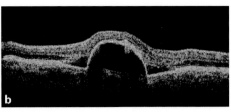

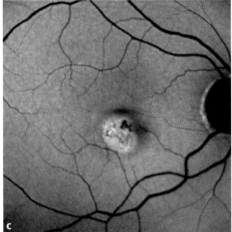

Fig. 13.3a–d Colour, optical coherence tomography, fluorescein angiogram, and corresponding fundus autofluorescence (FAF) image showing a large detachment of the retinal pigment epithelium with intermediate FAF signal and a surrounding halo of decreased autofluorescence signal in the presence of a RAP lesion

Fig 13.4 Variation of fundus autofluorescence (FAF) signal in the presence of a detachment of the retinal pigment epithelium over time. **a** Corresponding increased FAF and dark halo at baseline. **b** After 6 months, the autofluorescence signal decreases in the area of the detachment while the border becomes brightly autofluorescent

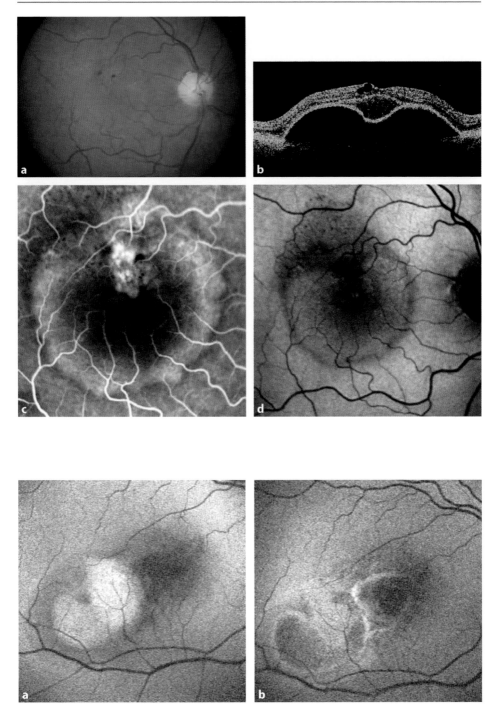

Fig. 13.5a–c Colour, indocyanine green angiogram, and corresponding fundus autofluorescence (FAF) image showing a detachment of the retinal pigment epithelium due to age-related macular degeneration, with decreased FAF signal over the lesion. Note the choroidal neovascular membrane at the inferior nasal part of the lesion

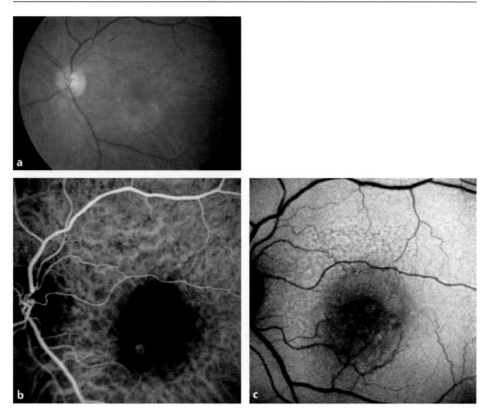

Fig. 13 6a–c Colour, fluorescein angiogram, and corresponding fundus auto-fluorescence (FAF) image of a detachment of the retinal pigment epithelium, showing a cartwheel pattern with corresponding hyperpigmented lines and diminished FAF signal between those lines

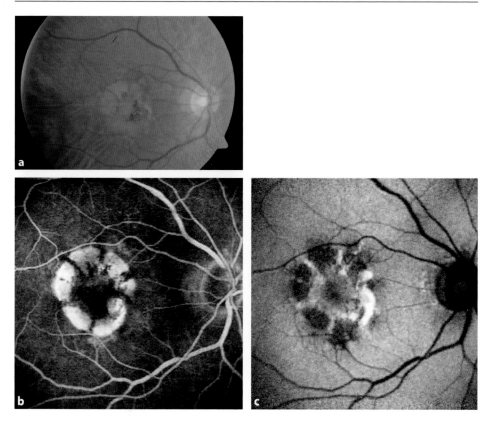

Age-Related Macular Degeneration IV — Choroidal Neovascularization (CNV)

14

Samantha S. Dandekar, Alan C. Bird

14.1
Introduction

Choroidal neovascularization (CNV) is a common cause of visual loss in patients with age-related macular degeneration (AMD) and represents the growth of subretinal new vessels in the macular region (Fig. 14.1) [1]. Central visual loss subsequently occurs following exudation and haemorrhage from the new vessel complex. It occurs in the setting of early age-related maculopathy, including drusen and pigment changes that consist of changes in the retinal pigment epithelium (RPE) and Bruch's membrane [8, 18, 20]. Blood vessels derived from the choroid extend through Bruch's membrane and into the sub-RPE space [9]. Lesions can be extrafoveal (edge >200 μm from the centre of the foveal avascular zone [FAZ]), juxtafoveal (1–199 μm from the FAZ), or subfoveal, where neovascularization occurs under the FAZ [3, 4].

The most recent theory of CNV development is that it occurs in response to the release of angiogenic stimuli from the RPE, including vascular endothelial growth factor (VEGF) [21, 30, 31]. Studies investigating the response of anti-VEGF treatments in CNV have had very encouraging results and further exemplify the importance of diagnosing lesions in their early stages [17, 19, 22]. The importance of the RPE in CNV development implies that fundus autofluorescence (FAF) imaging may be useful in its assessment. FAF imaging has allowed us to evaluate the integrity and metabolism of the RPE during ageing and ocular disease, its justification being based on the observations of Delori (see Chap. 2) [6, 25, 26, 32].

The assessment of the integrity of the RPE in CNV development may be important for two reasons. First, it may influence the behaviour of the choroidal new vessel complex, and second, visual acuity may be determined by whether the RPE maintains its physiological function [2, 33]. Unlike in geographic atrophy (GA), where FAF has been shown to be decreased in areas of RPE and photoreceptor loss and increased at the junctional zone (see Chap. 12), autofluorescence has been less well characterized in CNV [11].

14.2
FAF Findings in Early CNV

The distribution of FAF in patients with different stages of CNV development has been published and compared with fluorescein angiography [5, 7, 16, 23, 26–29]. Eyes with "recent-onset" CNV were found to have patches of "continuous" or "normal" autofluorescence corresponding to areas of hyperfluorescence on the comparative fluorescein angiograms (Fig. 14.2). This implied that RPE viability was preserved at least initially in CNV development. An increased FAF signal surrounding lesions appears to be less common in CNV compared with GA; it could be speculated that RPE lipofuscin may not play such an important role in the development of CNV.

The median visual acuity was found to be greater in the early CNV group, which may suggest that visual outcome is somewhat dependant on RPE preservation. A further finding from the study showed that the abnormal area according to the FAF image was statistically larger than that measured from the fluorescein image, implying that FAF imaging was better able to delineate the edge of CNV lesions [5].

In a subsequent study, intact foveal FAF correlated with visual acuity, size of the lesion, and symptom length, although no individual factor was predictive [24]. Intact FAF was also noted up to 20 months after diagnosis. The integrity of the RPE in the early stages would also support the hypothesis that VEGF and other growth factors are being released from viable RPE in the early stages of the disorder [13, 14].

14.3
FAF Findings in Late-Stage CNV

In the eyes with long-standing CNV, more areas of decreased AF were seen, implying non-viable RPE and lack of photoreceptor outer segment renewal (Fig. 14.3). It is likely that the areas of decreased FAF represent areas of RPE atrophy beneath the CNV scars in the late stages of disease [5].

It has also been shown that areas of increased FAF seen inferior to lesions are thought to be due to a gravitational effect of fluid tracking under the retina, similar to that seen in central serous retinopathy (Fig. 14.3, top row) [15]. Increased FAF signal has also been described around the edge of lesions that are thought to represent proliferation of RPE cells around the CNV (Fig. 14.1) [16].

14.4
FAF Findings in Relation to CNV Classification

The pattern of fluorescence on fluorescein angiography determines the classification of lesions as either classic (early, well-defined hyperfluorescence with late leakage and blurring of the margins; see Fig. 14.4) or occult (irregular, stippled hyperfluorescence or late leakage of undetermined source; see Fig. 14.5), based on the macular photocoagulation study definitions [3].

Histopathologic studies have shown that classic complexes have predominantly a subretinal fibrovascular component as opposed to most occult lesions that remain underneath the RPE [15]. This would imply that classic lesions are more likely to be visible on FAF imaging, although this does not always appear to be the case.

14.4.1
Classic CNV

A study by McBain et al. recently compared FAF imaging in classic and occult lesions, demonstrating differences between them [16]. Purely classic lesions showed low or decreased FAF signal at the site of the CNV, with a ring of increased FAF around some lesions (Figs. 14.1 and 14.4). The low signal area was thought to represent blockage of FAF caused by the CNV growing in the subretinal space, rather than direct damage to the RPE layer. It was felt that destruction of the RPE was unlikely, due to the homogeneity of the low signal seen in the images and given that all patients in the study had newly diagnosed CNV. The ring seen around some of the classic lesions was thought to represent proliferation of RPE cells around the CNV. According to Dandekar et al., it was felt that the increased FAF seen in some cases may be related to the phagocytosis of subretinal debris by macrophages [5].

14.4.2
Occult CNV

In occult lesions, a much more variable pattern of CNV was seen (Fig. 14.5) [5, 16]. This is not surprising given the more heterogeneous nature of such lesions. According to McBain et al., foci of decreased FAF were seen scattered within the lesion (Fig. 14.5, left column for similar appearance). These were felt to be due to small areas of RPE loss or damage caused by the chronic, more indolent lesions growing underneath the RPE. Areas of increased FAF were less frequently associated with the edge of occult lesions compared with predominantly classic lesions.

Other causes of decreased FAF signal in CNV lesions include blood, exudates, and fibrovascular scars (Figs. 14.3 and 14.5) [5]. Here, adjunctive tests such as ocular coherence tomography may help in interpreting FAF images and improving our understanding of the pathogenesis of CNV.

14.5
RPE Tears

RPE tears in the presence of AMD have been reported to occur in association with pigment epithelium detachment, either spontaneously or following therapeutic intervention (Fig. 14.6) [10]. FAF imaging may be helpful in establishing the diagnosis by visualization of the affected areas [12, 23]. Areas with RPE loss are characterised by a very low signal because of loss of lipofuscin and are sharply demarcated. The adjacent area with rolled-up RPE is characterised by heterogeneous signal of distinct increased FAF. Thus, the exact location of the tear can be delineated in most cases.

References

1. Bird, AC, Bressler, NM, Bressler, SB, et al. (1995) An international classification and grading system for age-related maculopathy and age-related macular degeneration. The International ARM Epidemiological Study Group. Surv Ophthalmol 39:367–374

2. Blaauwgeers, HG, Holtkamp, GM, Rutten, H, et al. (1999) Polarized vascular endothelial growth factor secretion by human retinal pigment epithelium and localization of vascular endothelial growth factor receptors on the inner choriocapillaris. Evidence for a trophic paracrine relation. Am J Pathol 155:421–428

3. Bressler, NM, Bressler, SB, Gragoudas, ES (1987) Clinical characteristics of choroidal neovascular membranes. Arch Ophthalmol 105:209–213

4. Chamberlin, JA, Bressler, NM, Bressler, SB, et al. (1989) The use of fundus photographs and fluorescein angiograms in the identification and treatment of choroidal neovascularization in the Macular Photocoagulation Study. The Macular Photocoagulation Study Group. Ophthalmology 96:1526–1534

5. Dandekar, SS, Jenkins, SA, Peto, T, et al. (2005) Autofluorescence imaging of choroidal neovascularization due to age-related macular degeneration. Arch Ophthalmol 123:1507–1513

6. Delori, FC, Dorey, CK, Staurenghi, G, et al. (1995) In vivo fluorescence of the ocular fundus exhibits retinal pigment epithelium lipofuscin characteristics. Invest Ophthalmol Vis Sci 36:718–729

7. Framme, C, Bunse, A, Sofroni, R, et al. (2006) Fundus autofluorescence before and after photodynamic therapy for choroidal neovascularization secondary to age-related macular degeneration. Ophthalmic Surg Lasers Imaging 37:406–414

8. Green, WR (1999) Histopathology of age-related macular degeneration. Mol Vis 5:27

9. Green, WR, Engel, C (1992) Age-related macular degeneration: histopathologic studies: the 1992 Lorenz E. Zimmermann Lecture. Ophthalmology 100:1519–1535

10. Holz, G, Pauleikhoff, D, Spaide, RF, Bird, AC (2004) Age-related macular degeneration. Springer, Berlin

11. Holz, FG, Bellmann, C, Margaritidis, M, et al. (1999) Patterns of increased in vivo fundus autofluorescence in the junctional zone of geographic atrophy of the retinal pigment epithelium associated with age-related macular degeneration. Graefes Arch Clin Exp Ophthalmol 237:145–152

12. Karadimas, P, Paleokastritis, G P, Bouzas, EA (2006) Fundus autofluorescence imaging findings in retinal pigment epithelial tear. Eur J Ophthalmol 16:767–769

13. Kliffen, M, Sharma, HS, Mooy, CM, et al. (1997) Increased expression of angiogenic growth factors in age-related maculopathy. Br J Ophthalmol 81:154–162

14. Kvanta, A, Algvere, PV, Berglin, L, Seregard, S (1996) Subfoveal fibrovascular membranes in age-related macular degeneration express vascular endothelial growth factor. Invest Ophthalmol Vis Sci 37:1929–1934

15. Lafaut, BA, Bartz-Schmidt, KU, Vanden Broecke, C, et al. (2000) Clinicopathological correlation in exudative age related macular degeneration: histological differentiation between classic and occult choroidal neovascularization. Br J Ophthalmol 84:239–243

16. McBain, VA, Townend, J, Lois, N (2006) Fundus autofluorescence in exudative age-related macular degeneration. Br J Ophthalmol

17. Michels, S, Rosenfeld, PJ, Puliafito, CA, et al. (2005) Systemic bevacizumab (Avastin) therapy for neovascular age-related macular degeneration twelve-week results of an uncontrolled open-label clinical study. Ophthalmology 112:1035–1047

18. Pauleikhoff, D, Harper, CA, Marshall, J, Bird, AC (1990) Aging changes in Bruch's membrane. A histochemical and morphologic study. Ophthalmology 97:171–178

19. Rosenfeld, PJ, Brown, DM, Heier, JS, et al. (2006) Ranibizumab for neovascular age-related macular degeneration. N Engl J Med 355:1419–1431

20. Sarks, SH (1976) Ageing and degeneration in the macular region: a clinico-pathological study. Br J Ophthalmol 60:324–341

21. Schwesinger, C, Yee, C, Rohan, RM, et al. (2001) Intrachoroidal neovascularization in transgenic mice overexpressing vascular endothelial growth factor in the retinal pigment epithelium. Am J Pathol 158:1161–1172

22. Spaide, RF, Laud, K, Fine, HF, et al. (2006) Intravitreal bevacizumab treatment of choroidal neovascularization secondary to age-related macular degeneration. Retina 26:383–390

23. Spital, G, Radermacher, M, Muller, C, et al. (1998) [Autofluorescence characteristics of lipofuscin components in different forms of late senile macular degeneration]. Klin Monatsbl Augenheilkd 213:23–31

24. Vaclavik, V, Dandekar, SS, Vujosevic, S, et al. (2006) Integrity of the retinal pigment epithelium (RPE) in early choroidal neovascularization (CNV) in age-related macular disease (AMD). Oxford Congress (poster presentation), July 1, 2006

25. von Rückmann, A, Fitzke, FW, Bird, AC (1995) Distribution of fundus autofluorescence with a scanning laser ophthalmoscope. Br J Ophthalmol 79:407–412

26. von Rückmann, A, Fitzke, FW, Bird, AC (1997) Fundus autofluorescence in age-related macular disease imaged with a laser scanning ophthalmoscope. Invest Ophthalmol Vis Sci 38:478–486

27. von Rückmann, A, Schmidt, KG, Fitzke, FW, et al. (1998) [Studies of the distribution of lipofuscin in the retinal pigment epithelium using high-resolution TV laser scanning ophthalmoscopy]. Ophthalmologe 95:699–705

28. von Rückmann, A, Schmidt, KG, Fitzke, FW, et al. (1998) [Fundus autofluorescence in patients with hereditary macular dystrophies, malattia leventinese, familial dominant and aged-related drusen]. Klin Monatsbl Augenheilkd 213:81–86

29. von Rückmann, A, Schmidt, KG, Fitzke, FW, et al. (1998) [Dynamics of accumulation and degradation of lipofuscin in retinal pigment epithelium in senile macular degeneration]. Klin Monatsbl Augenheilkd 213:32–37

30. Wada, M, Ogata, N, Otsuji, T, Uyama, M (1999) Expression of vascular endothelial growth factor and its receptor (KDR/flk-1) mRNA in experimental choroidal neovascularization. Curr Eye Res 18:203–213

31. Wells, JA, Murthy, R, Chibber, R, et al. (1996) Levels of vascular endothelial growth factor are elevated in the vitreous of patients with subretinal neovascularization. Br J Ophthalmol 80:363–366

32. Wing, GL, Blanchard, GC, Weiter, JJ (1978) The topography and age relationship of lipofuscin concentration in the retinal pigment epithelium. Invest Ophthalmol Vis Sci 17:601–607

33. Yamagishi, K, Ohkuma, H, Itagaki, T, et al. (1988) [Implication of retinal pigment epithelium on experimental subretinal neovascularization in the developmental stage]. Nippon Ganka Gakkai Zasshi 92:1629–1636

Fig. 14.1 Colour, fluorescein angiogram, and fundus autofluorescence (FAF) images of two eyes with choroidal neovascularization (CNV). *Left column:* CNV lesion with a few small exudates superiorly and haemorrhage at the nasal border. Note that blood and exudate appear dark on FAF imaging. The lesion itself, which leaks on fluorescein angiography, appears to be of background FAF intensity, implying an intact retinal pigment epithelium (RPE) layer. *Right column:* The edge of this subfoveal CNV lesion is seen more clearly on the fluorescein image, but the abnormal area on FAF imaging appears to be larger than that seen on fluorescein angiography [5]. Note the increased FAF around both lesions, thought to be suggestive of proliferation of RPE cells around the CNV [16]

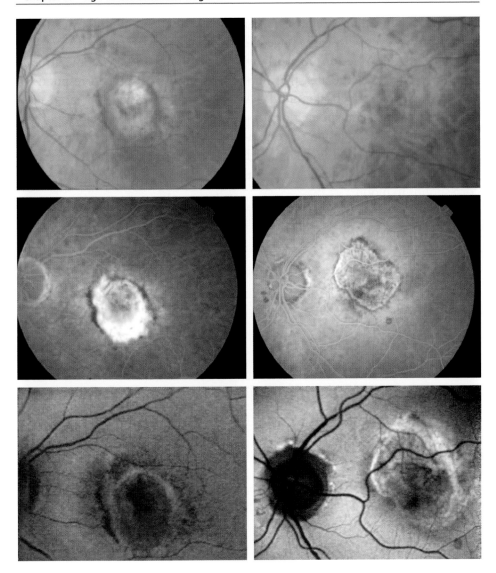

Fig. 14.2 Colour, fluorescein angiogram, and fundus autofluorescence (FAF) images of two eyes with early-stage choroidal neovascularization (CNV). *Left column:* Early CNV lesion inferiorly with a small area of geographic atrophy superiorly. Note that the area that fluoresces within the CNV corresponds to an area of "normal" or "background" FAF intensity. The area of decreased autofluorescence represents an area of atrophy. *Right column:* The majority of this newly diagnosed CNV lesion corresponds to areas with "normal" FAF intensity, with a band of increased FAF signal adjacent to the area of hyperfluorescence seen on the fluorescein angiogram. The reduced FAF signal around the edge corresponds to blood

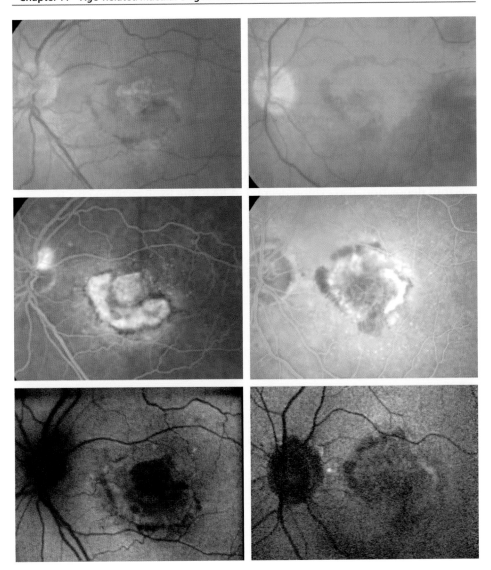

Fig. 14.3 Colour and fundus autofluorescence (FAF) images of three eyes with late-stage choroidal neovascularization (CNV). *Top row:* Late-stage CNV lesion with an increased FAF signal below the lesion, representing a gravitational effect of fluid tracking beneath the retina. *Middle row:* Disciform scar secondary to CNV with corresponding areas of decreased FAF, implying retinal pigment epithelium (RPE) cell and photoreceptor loss. Increased autofluorescence signal may represent macrophages or proliferation of RPE cells at the edge of the lesion. *Bottom row:* End-stage disease with widespread areas of reduced FAF, implying atrophy and RPE loss. Note that areas with pigment migration and melanin deposition also exhibit decreased FAF due to absorption effects

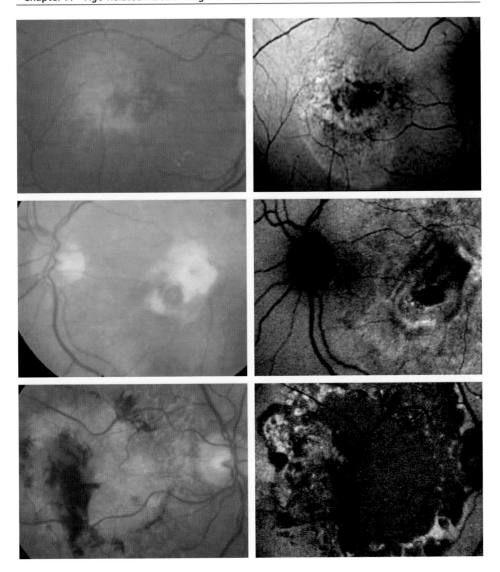

Fig. 14.4 Colour, fluorescein angiogram, and fundus autofluorescence (FAF) images of two eyes with classic choroidal neovascularization (CNV). *Left column:* Predominantly classic CNV lesion with near "normal" or background FAF signal, implying preserved retinal pigment epithelium (RPE) function. This lesion does not show a surrounding area of increased FAF. *Right column:* Classic lesion with some increased FAF signal towards the edge of the lesion. This may also represent proliferation of RPE cells. Images courtesy of V. Vaclavik

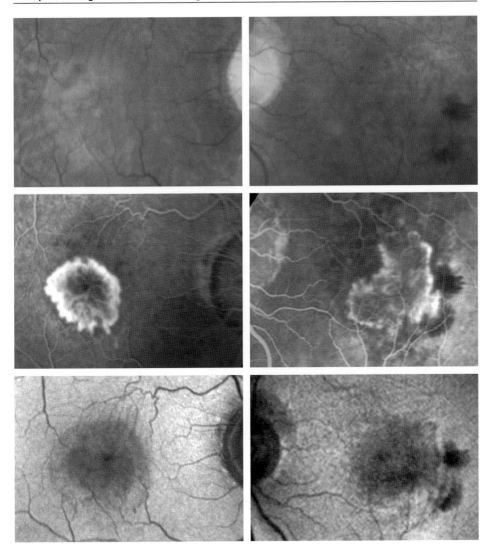

Fig. 14.5 Colour, fluorescein angiogram, and fundus autofluorescence (FAF) images of two eyes with occult choroidal neovascularization (CNV). *Left column:* Occult CNV lesion with a heterogeneous appearance on the FAF image. *Right column:* Occult lesion with areas of decreased signal corresponding to blood and possibly to areas of retinal pigment epithelium loss (temporal part)

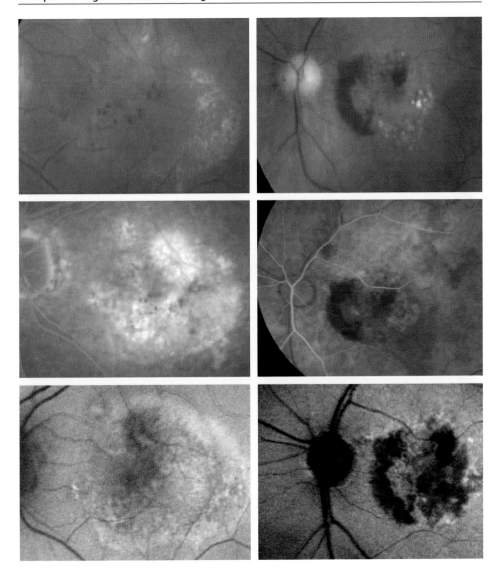

Fig. 14.6 Retinal pigment epithelium tear following development of choroidal neovascularization secondary to age-related macular degeneration, illustrated by fundus photograph, fundus autofluorescence image, and fluorescein angiogram (early and late phases)

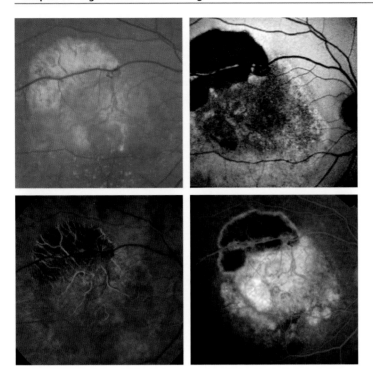

Idiopathic Macular Telangiectasia

Peter Charbel Issa, Hendrik P.N. Scholl,
Hans-Martin Helb, Frank G. Holz

15

15.1
Introduction

Idiopathic macular telangiectasia (IMT; also known as idiopathic parafoveal telangiectasis) is a descriptive term for different disease entities presenting with telangiectatic alterations of the juxtafoveolar capillary network with a predominant location temporal to the fovea [1–3, 5]. IMT is distinct from similar vascular alterations that may develop secondary to retinal vein occlusion, vasculitis, diabetes, carotid occlusive disease, or radiation therapy.

The most commonly used classification to date was introduced by Gass and Blodi in 1993 and comprises three types [3]. Type 1 predominantly presents in males with unilateral telangiectasia and macular edema. Type 2 is usually bilateral with atrophy of the neurosensory retina. Type 3 is extremely rare and is characterized by progressive obliteration of the perifoveal capillary network.

As outlined in Chap. 5, macular pigment optical density (MPOD) can be assessed by subtraction of two autofluorescence images obtained at different wavelengths (488 nm and 514 nm) with a confocal scanning laser ophthalmoscope (Fig. 15.1c,d). Application of this method in IMT has recently led to the identification of a previously unknown phenomenon of depletion of macular pigment in type 2 IMT [4]. The underlying mechanism is unknown, although it may be speculated that impaired trafficking and/or storage of lutein and zeaxanthin may play a role. The finding may point towards a dysfunction of cells participating in this process. Therefore, it was speculated that the vascular alterations in type 2 IMT may represent a secondary phenomenon. Interestingly, depletion of macular pigment occurs in type 2 IMT but not type 1. It is therefore also of diagnostic importance to perform fundus autofluorescence (FAF) imaging when the distinction by other diagnostic means may not be obvious.

15.2
FAF in Type 1 Idiopathic Macular Telangiectasia

Type 1 idiopathic macular telangiectasia (type 1 IMT) mostly occurs unilaterally and is considered to be a developmental anomaly. Characteristic visible aneurysmatic capillary changes are accompanied by a cystic macular edema with exudation (Fig. 15.1a, b). FAF imaging may show an increased signal that may be explained by a reduced MPOD due to retinal tissue defects in the area with cystoid changes (Fig. 15.1c,d,f). However, overall the distribution is normal, with the highest MPOD in the fovea and attenuation towards the periphery.

15.3
FAF in Type 2 Idiopathic Macular Telangiectasia

Type 2 IMT is the most common form of IMT and occurs without obvious gender predilection. It typically becomes symptomatic in the 5th or 6th decade of life. Because of a cumulated occurrence within families and monozygotic twins, a genetic background has been suggested [1].

The major vascular abnormality appears to mainly affect the deep parafoveal capillary network. Early-phase fluorescein angiography reveals ectatic-appearing parafoveal capillaries (Fig. 15.2a). A diffuse parafoveal hyperfluorescence is seen in late-phase fluorescein angiography, predominantly located in the deep neurosensory retina and/or subretinal space (Fig. 15.2b). There is no accompanying cystoid edema but rather an atrophic neurosensory retina. Ophthalmoscopically, superficial crystalline deposits and, in later stages, intraretinal pigment clumping may occur (Fig. 15.2c). Funduscopically, a characteristic parafoveal loss of retinal transparency ("retinal greying") may be observed (Fig. 15.2c). Moreover, there is an increased reflectance in confocal blue reflectance imaging within the area of retinal greying (Fig. 15.2d).

MPOD is typically reduced in the macular area (Fig. 15.2f), and the area of depletion largely corresponds to angiographic late-phase hyperfluorescence (Fig. 15.2b) and increased confocal blue reflectance (Fig. 15.2d). Possibly, the latter is a secondary phenomenon to the decreased macular pigment. FAF may be only minimally altered in very early disease stages (Fig. 15.3b). However, in later disease stages the FAF signal is typically grossly abnormal. (Fig. 15.3d, f). When intraretinal pigment clumping has occurred, FAF may show a reduced signal due to a blockade phenomenon (Fig. 15.2e).

References

1. Charbel Issa P, Scholl HPN, Helb HM, et al. (2007) Macular telangiectasia. In: Holz FG, Spaide RF (eds). Medical retina. Springer, Heidelberg, 183–197

2. Gass JD, Blodi BA (1993) Idiopathic juxtafoveolar retinal telangiectasis. Update of classification and follow-up study. Ophthalmology 100:1536–1546

3. Helb HM, Charbel Issa P, Pauleikhoff D, Scholl HPN, Holz FG (2006) Macular pigment density and distribution in patients with macular telangiectasia. Invest Ophthalmol Vis Sci:#5701/B795 [ARVO abstract]

4. Yannuzzi LA, Bardal AM, Freund KB, et al. (2006) Idiopathic macular telangiectasia. Arch Ophthalmol 124:450-460

Fig. 15.1 a,b Early- and late-phase fluorescein angiogram of an eye with type 1 idiopathic macular telangiectasia (IMT). The funduscopically visible aneurysms show a marked leakage. Late-phase leakage fills a large foveal cyst. **c,d** Fundus autofluorescence image at excitation wavelengths of 488 nm (**c**) and 514 nm (**d**). The increased signal in the area of the cystoid foveal changes might be explained by the lack of macular pigment (**f**). **e,f** Macular pigment optical density distribution in the healthy right eye (**e**) and in the left eye with type 1 IMT (**f**)

Fig. 15.2 Early- and late-phase fluorescein angiography, colour fundus photograph, confocal blue reflectance image, fundus autofluorescence (FAF) image, and macular pigment optical density in an eye with a late disease stage of type 2 idiopathic macular telangiectasia. There is an increased signal in FAF imaging in proximity to the intraretinal pigment clumping temporal to the fovea (**e**). The lack of macular pigment (**f**) is topographically related to the diffuse hyperfluorescence in late-phase fluorescein angiography (**b**), to the parafoveal loss of transparency (**c**), and to the increased parafoveal confocal blue reflectance (**d**)

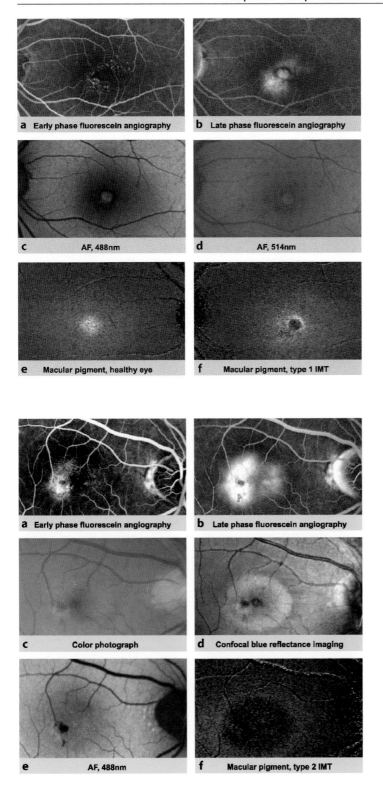

a   Early phase fluorescein angiography

b   Late phase fluorescein angiography

c   AF, 488nm

d   AF, 514nm

e   Macular pigment, healthy eye

f   Macular pigment, type 1 IMT

a   Early phase fluorescein angiography

b   Late phase fluorescein angiography

c   Color photograph

d   Confocal blue reflectance imaging

e   AF, 488nm

f   Macular pigment, type 2 IMT

Fig. 15.3 Late-phase fluorescein angiograms (*left*) and fundus autofluorescence (FAF) images (*right*) in the eyes of three different patients with type 2 idiopathic macular telangiectasia. **a,b** An early disease stage. In contrast to normal subjects (see Chap. 7), FAF imaging shows no levels of decreased intensities in the fovea. **c–f** Later disease stages. There is even an increased FAF signal predominantly temporal to the fovea

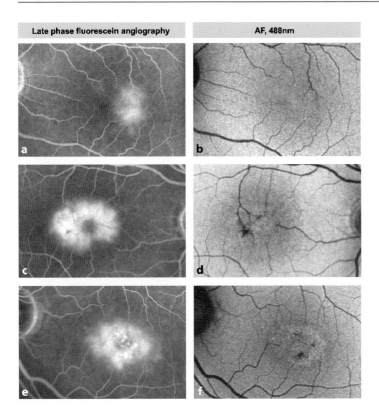

Chorioretinal Inflammatory Disorders

16

Richard F. Spaide

Introduction

Autofluorescence photography complements other methods of imaging the ocular fundus. The amount of autofluorescence is governed by the amount of fluorophores in any given area in the fundus. Inflammation can alter the amounts of fluorophores during acute phases, and the injured tissue behaves according to observable rules during resolution. Choroidal neovascularization (CNV) associated with intraocular inflammation is a common complication, and this secondary CNV produces characteristic autofluorescence findings. By observing autofluorescence characteristics, we can estimate the extent of damage, diagnose sequelae such as secondary CNV, learn more about the inflammatory process in question, and possibly anticipate future problems caused by disease. However, autofluorescence photography is almost always used with alternate means of imaging, such as optical coherence tomography (OCT), fluorescein angiography, and indocyanine green (ICG) angiography. Autofluorescence photography contributes information that alternate methods of imaging cannot and does so through a noninvasive means.

Interpretation of the autofluorescence findings of ocular inflammatory diseases requires some additional considerations to those used for interpreting autofluorescence images of degenerations and aging. These considerations arose from observation of fundus autofluorescence over time for a variety of inflammatory diseases. There is almost no published information concerning what inflammation does in the creation or processing of fluorophores in the eye, limiting available information to cumulated experience from clinical evaluation of cases. The pathophysiologic changes that occur with intraocular inflammation follow a stepwise orderly sequence. The autofluorescence changes also vary by the size of the lesion. Smaller inflammatory lesions affecting the retinal pigment epithelium (RPE), such as those seen with multifocal choroiditis and panuveitis (MCP), are often just hypofluorescent when first detected. Inflammatory lesions affecting larger areas of the RPE usually have a more complex appearance, which varies by the age of the lesion.

Acute inflammatory changes cause a color change at the level of the RPE, which is associated with a varying amount of thickening at the level of the RPE as well (Fig. 16.1). There may be increased autofluorescence in acute phases, but several inflammatory diseases have increased autofluorescence in the subacute phases. This increase in autofluorescence may be due to a number of factors. It is possible that the size and number of fluorophore content of the RPE cells is altered by inflammation. Certainly, inflammation induces a number of pro-oxidative pathways, which may increase the amount of fluorophores present. Hypertrophy and reactive hyperplasia of the RPE may increase the thickness of the RPE, contributing to the formation of autofluorescence. Associated with the increase in autofluorescence is an increase in visible pigmentation in the RPE. The areas of RPE with increased pigmentation also show increased autofluorescence. On ophthalmoscopy, these pigmented areas are yellowish-brown in color. The pathways in cell metabolism leading to lipofuscin are intertwined with those leading to melanin formation [11, 14, 18, 21–23, 33]. Stressed RPE cells appear to fuse phagosomes containing ingested outer segments with melanosomes as a pathway of metabolism [22]. In addition, oxidation of melanin within RPE cells leads to the generation of fluorophores having absorption and emission spectra similar to lipofuscin [14, 21].

With time, the areas start to become thinner, and they appear to shrink in a lateral sense. The inflammatory lesion retracts centripetally, leaving a surrounding gap void of fluorescing RPE cells. This gap appears as a transmission defect during fluorescein angiography because of the lack of pigment, and it appears very dark during autofluorescence photography because of the lack of fluorophores. During the resolution stages of inflammation, the pigment in the lesion becomes slate-grey. With this change in color comes a decrease in the amount of autofluorescence visible. Slate or neutral grey-black areas frequently have an absence of autofluorescence. The formerly dark halo around inflammatory lesions may show autofluorescent dots, possibly indicating a repopulation of the zone devoid of functional RPE cells.

Secondary CNV is almost always classic, corresponding to what Grossniklaus and Gass classified as type 2 CNV [9]. This variant of CNV grows on the inner side of the RPE monolayer but is frequently enveloped in reactive hyperplastic RPE cells. Secondary CNV is often easy to recognize by autofluorescence photography because the surrounding hyperplastic RPE is hyperautofluorescent and neatly outlines the neovascularization. This hyperautofluorescence persists for years after the CNV has formed. Following treatment, CNV may contract and leave a zone of absent RPE in a manner similar to inflammatory lesions.

16.2
Acute Posterior Multifocal Placoid Pigment Epitheliopathy

Gass [8] described three young women who developed acute, but transient, loss of visual acuity associated with multiple yellow-white placoid lesions at the level of the RPE. The disorder was presumed to primarily involve the RPE and was named with the descriptive term of acute posterior multifocal placoid pigment epitheliopathy (APMPPE) [8]. Soon after the original description, Deutman and associates [2] hypothesized that an acute inflammation of the choriocapillaris was the initial incident in APMPPE and that the RPE changes were a subsequent manifestation. ICG angiography [12] and OCT [15] showed additional information, but neither of these methods of imaging primarily evaluates the RPE. APMPPE has been seen in association with a diverse number of diseases, and this diversity raises the question of how multiple isolated patches of the RPE could be affected independently by these afflictions without first involving the choroidal vasculature. In addition, APMPPE is associated with signs of vasculitis, not only in the choroid [28] but in other organ systems as well.

In the acute phases of APMPPE, more lesions are visible by either fluorescein angiography or ophthalmoscopy than are visible by autofluorescence photography [29] (Figs. 16.2–16.4). Many of these hypofluorescent areas were not associated with observable changes of the RPE, suggesting the presence of choriocapillaris perfusion defects. In the subacute phases there is prominent late staining of APMPPE lesions during fluorescein angiography. These same lesions have autofluorescence abnormalities that match the size and shape of the areas seen in later phases of the angiogram. Follow-up examination shows that many lesions develop increased pigmentation centrally with a depigmented halo. These same lesions have shown concurrent late staining during fluorescein angiography and prominent autofluorescence findings. The depigmented halo appeared to show increased fluorescence during fluorescein angiography and decreased, almost absent, autofluorescence. The central portions of the lesions, which appeared to have increased pigment, were intensely autofluorescent but showed blocking during fluorescein angiography.

The increased pigmentation of the central portion of the lesions with areas of depigmentation is not uncommon in healing APMPPE lesions. Although altered pigmentation of the RPE is common after injury or inflammation, the pattern seen in this patient with APMPPE (Figs. 16.2–16.4) suggests there may be a possible pathophysiologic explanation. The areas of decreased pigmentation with increased fluorescence and decreased autofluorescence suggest atrophy or absence of functional RPE cells. Increased pigmentation and increased autofluorescence can result from increased content of pigment within RPE cells or thickening or duplication of the RPE. Given the finding of increased pigmentation and autofluorescence centrally with a depigmented hypoautofluorescent surround, it is possible that with healing of the lesions there was a centripetal contraction of each placoid lesion with retraction of the edges inward. This would create the hypopigmented surround in the process. The autofluorescence changes seen in this patient lagged behind the appearance of the placoid lesions, which in turn did not seem as numerous as the choroidal abnormalities as determined by fluorescein and ICG angiography. The implication of these findings is that the RPE is affected secondarily to the choroidal changes, and the RPE undergoes alterations well after the choroid is affected.

16.3
Acute Syphilitic Posterior Placoid Chorioretinitis

Syphilis causes various patterns of inflammation in the anterior chamber, vitreous, retina, and optic nerve, often mimicking other diseases. Patients with secondary syphilis may develop an acute, yellow placoid lesion in the macular region [5] (Figs. 16.5–16.8). The appearance of the yellow placoid lesion has been likened to those seen in APMPPE. The level of involvement of acute syphilitic posterior placoid chorioretinopathy (ASPPC) has been attributed to alterations in the retina and choroid. ASPPC is an uncommon condition in patients with secondary syphilis. The patients have acute vision dysfunction in one eye and yellow-white placoid lesion in the macular area [1, 5, 34]; these placoid lesion findings are more prominent at the outer border of the lesion. Fluorescein staining and increased autofluorescence are more evident where the lesion has a greater yellow color. With treatment, the yellow color, opacification of the retina, increased autofluorescence, and staining by fluorescein angiography resolve.

ASPPC shares similarities to APMPPE in that both conditions can cause yellowish plaque-like changes in the posterior pole [16]. There are important differences in appearance, and probably in pathophysiology. ASPPC usually causes a solitary yellow placoid lesion that has a more prominent color and opacification at its outer borders. The autofluorescence abnormalities are confined only to the placoid region. One patient had small zones of blocked fluorescence on fluorescein angiography due to clumps of yellowish material that was hyperautofluorescent. These blocked areas of fluorescence mimicked the appearance of focal areas of abnormal perfusion, which has been reported previously in a patient, but none of our patients showed signs of choroidal vascular perfusion abnormalities. In APMPPE there are many areas of decreased perfusion of the choriocapillaris seen early in the fluorescein angiogram, most of which are associated with yellowish placoid changes [5]. These perfusion defects are about half of a disc area in size or are multiples of that quantum size. Only some of the yellow lesions show autofluorescent abnormalities.

It appears that ASPPC affects the RPE and possibly the outer retina. The yellow color in both ASPPC and APMPPE may be due to involvement of the RPE. In the case of APMPPE this appears to be secondary to primary choriocapillaris involvement, something that does not appear to occur in early ASPPC. In addition to the inflammatory changes in ASPPC, there is an increase in autofluorescence, which may be due to the accumulation of lipofuscin in the RPE or to imperfect phagocytosis and processing of photoreceptor outer segments in the acute phases of the disease. Accumulation of the outer segments in the subretinal space may explain the yellowish clumps of material seen in case 1 (Fig. 16.5). Decreased phagocytosis of outer segments with accumulation of subretinal material has been seen in ocular tumors [32], central serous chorioretinopathy [26], and vitelliform macular dystrophy [27].

16.4
Multifocal Choroiditis and Panuveitis

Multifocal choroiditis and panuveitis (MCP) is an inflammatory disease primarily affecting myopic women in their 3rd–5th decades of life [3, 17]. The hallmarks of the disease are small round chorioretinal scars, scattered or in linear aggregates; peripapillary scarring; a high propensity to develop choroidal neovascularization; and periodic episodes of clinically evident intraocular inflammation [3]. This inflammation is usually evident as cells in the vitreous and infiltrates in the choroid. Retinal vasculitis and optic disc edema are less commonly seen. Presumed ocular histoplasmosis syndrome (POHS) also causes somewhat similar findings, with the exception that POHS is generally found in endemic regions, causes five or fewer chorioretinal scars, and is not associated with clinically evident intraocular inflammation [25].

Indocyanine green angiography imaging of patients with MCP shows hypofluorescent spots within the choroid, and the number of these hypofluorescent spots often exceeds that of the chorioretinal scars seen by ophthalmoscopy [24] (Figs. 16.9 and 16.10). This finding implies that there may be abnormalities in the choroid of patients with MCP that cannot be directly seen by ophthalmoscopy. An important cellular layer separating the retina and choroid is the RPE, abnormalities of which may have significant impact on visual function. Gross abnormalities of the RPE can be seen with ophthalmoscopy or fluorescein angiography, but many abnormalities of the RPE are most efficiently imaged with autofluorescence photography [31].

Autofluorescence photography of MCP demonstrates several interesting findings [10]. Clinically visible chorioretinal scars are hypoautofluorescent. This can be expected because if there were enough inflammation to damage the choroid and retina, the RPE would likely be damaged as well. However, autofluorescence photography often shows many more times the number of hypoautofluorescent spots than the number of chorioretinal scars. The hypoautofluorescent spots are very small, and clinically visible scars appear to be composed of multiple smaller hypoautofluorescent spots. Later development of visible chorioretinal spots has occurred in areas occupied by the hypoautofluorescent spots seen by autofluorescence imaging. Thus autofluorescence photography appears to show areas of RPE damage from MCP that are more numerous and extensive than what the choroidal scars would indicate. It is possible that the hypoautofluorescent spots at the level of the RPE are remnants of inflammation spilling over from the choroid that was sufficient to cause RPE damage but not any significant choroidal changes. But it is also possible that multifocal choroiditis also primarily affects the RPE. Patients with MCP have additional areas affected by inflammation in that they can have retinal vasculitis, optic disc edema, frank optic neuropathy, and vitreous cells. The disease is named after the clinically evident change—that of multiple areas of choroidal involvement. In any case, the amount of retinal pigment epithelial damage seems to exceed the visible change within the choroid, suggesting some of the visual morbidity of MCP may be due to RPE damage.

Secondary choroidal neovascularization is visible as a butterfly-shaped area of hyperautofluorescence. The borders of the autofluorescence show prominent attachments to hypoautofluorescent MCP scars. The hyperautofluorescence of past CNV persists despite subsequent treatment. Of interest is the finding of small hyperautofluorescent spots or rings in the vicinity of MCP scars. CNV arising within ocular histoplasmosis scars has been theorized to occur. Diagnosis of CNV within histoplasmosis scars is difficult because of the small size, lack of hemorrhage, and the fact that the vessels do not necessarily grow beyond the margins of the scar. The same process appears to occur in MCP, in which patients develop small areas of CNV within MCP scars.

16.5
Acute Zonal Occult Outer Retinopathy

Gass [6, 7] described a rare syndrome of acute loss of one or more zones of what were believed to be outer retinal function, photopsias, and visual field defects frequently involving the blind spot, with minimal changes visible in the fundus, and named the disorder acute zonal occult outer retinopathy (AZOOR). Most of the affected patients were female and many had evidence of autoimmune diseases [4]. Affected patients had scotomata with associated photopsias, and some experienced a chronic smoldering disease with extensive field loss and decreased central visual acuity. AZOOR was described by Gass as being a superset of other inflammatory retinochoroidopathies, many of which are referred to as the white dot syndromes [7]. He noted that many of the diseases occur in women with a prior viral syndrome; that they caused visual field loss and photopsias and affected the outer retina; and that patients had developed more than one white dot syndrome, something that would not be expected by chance alone. He suspected that many of the white dot syndromes were caused by the same entity and thus could be grouped under the term "AZOOR complex." Jampol and Becker hypothesized a common genetic hypothesis of autoimmune and inflammatory disease. This hypothesis is an outgrowth of Becker's ideas that patients may have relatively common non-disease-specific genes that predispose them to autoimmune or inflammatory diseases. Environmental triggers interact with the explicit genetic make-up of the patient to produce a given likelihood of developing an inflammatory disease of a specific type. Because the genes altering the susceptibility are common and can be assorted, one or more seemingly disparate autoimmune diseases can arise in the same patient. Jampol and Becker [13] stated that because it is difficult to prove specific infectious causes for these diseases, a debate about infectious versus autoimmune etiology is not meaningful. Over the years, these two points of view, neither of which can explain all aspects of the disease and which are not mutually exclusive, have been framed as a pseudodebate.

The autofluorescent findings in AZOOR are based on a limited number of patients, largely because AZOOR is a rare disease (Figs. 16.11–16.14). In one published case the peripapillary distribution of AZOOR was evident [30]. The patient had a region of RPE atrophy as evidenced by subtle depigmentation and a transmission defect during fluorescein angiography. The patient also appeared to have atrophy of the choriocapillaris in the same zonal region during ICG angiography. Autofluorescence photography showed that the outer border was intensely autofluorescent, consistent with the presence of lipofuscin, and that the central area of the lesion was hypoautofluorescent, consistent with atrophy of the RPE. The patient had visual field abnormalities in the eye consistent with the location and size of the autofluorescence abnormality. Over a 2.5-year follow-up the patient had decreasing frequency of photopsias. The outer border appeared to have less intense hyperautofluorescence over time. (Other patients with AZOOR have had similar resolution of the hyperautofluorescent outer border as the disease waned.)

These findings suggest that the AZOOR syndrome caused an area of RPE cell death with lipofuscin-laden cells at the border of the expanding lesion in this patient. A secondary consequence of the RPE atrophy appeared to be choriocapillaris atrophy as evidenced by hypofluorescence in the involved area during ICG angiography that did not appear to involve the fluorescence of the underlying larger choroidal vessels. Application of these imaging techniques to greater numbers of patients with AZOOR may help appraise the true nature of the syndrome and the seemingly disparate constituent manifestations that have been attributed to this condition.

There have been patients who presented with findings typical of multiple evanescent white dot syndrome, which does not have striking autofluorescence findings, but later developed autofluorescent findings typical of AZOOR (Fig. 16.15). This progression of disease would be difficult to explain by stating that a patient had a common genetic predisposition to MEWDS or AZOOR, since they sequentially show signs of both. Other patients have had signs of having MEWDS and MCP [35], or MEWDS and acute macular neuroretinopathy [36]. Patients with multifocal choroiditis and visual field loss in excess to what would be expected by ophthalmoscopy have been reported, but patients with MCP can develop acute changes in their visual field that are responsive to corticosteroid therapy. Autofluorescence photography has demonstrated a peripapillary loss of autofluorescence suggestive of past AZOOR in one patient with MCP.

16.6
Birdshot Chorioretinopathy

Birdshot chorioretinopathy is an idiopathic, chronic, bilateral, chorioretinal inflammatory disease characterized by cream-colored ovoid spots at the level of the inner choroid (Figs. 16.16 and 16.17) [19, 20]. Eventually, the disease can cause loss of visual field, color vision abnormalities, nyctalopia, and central visual acuity loss. Birdshot chorioretinopathy causes two main types of lesions: a cream-colored inflammatory lesion and a depigmented lesion that can appear similar to the inflammatory lesion. The depigmented lesion is a burned-out scar caused by the inflammation. Larger choroidal vessels can be seen coursing under the depigmented lesions. Autofluorescent abnormalities are usually associated with the depigmented lesions, while the early lesions do not necessarily cause autofluorescent abnormalities. Birdshot chorioretinopathy can eventually cause widespread damage in the fundus, with large areas of RPE being affected.

References

1. Bellmann G, Holz FG, Breitbart A, Volcker HE. Bilateral acute syphilitische posteriore plakoide chorioretinopathy (ASPPC). Ophthalmologe. 1999;96:522–528

2. Deutman AF, Oosterhuis JA, Boen-Tan TN, and Aan De Kerk AL. Acute posterior multifocal placoid pigment epitheliopathy. Pigment epitheliopathy or choriocapillaritis? Brit J Ophthal 1972;56:863–874

3. Dreyer, RF and DJ Gass. Multifocal choroiditis and panuveitis. A syndrome that mimics ocular histoplasmosis. Arch Ophthalmol 1984;102:1776–1784

4. Gass JD, Agarwal A, Scott IU. Acute zonal occult outer retinopathy: a long-term follow-up study. Am J Ophthalmol 2002;134:329–339

5. Gass JD, Braunstein RA, Chenoweth RG. Acute syphilitic posterior placoid chorioretinitis. Ophthalmology 1990;97:1288–1297

6. Gass JD. Acute zonal occult outer retinopathy. Donders Lecture: The Netherlands Ophthalmological Society, Maastricht, Holland, June 19, 1992. J Clin Neuroophthalmol. 1993; 13:79–97

7. Gass JD. Are acute zonal occult outer retinopathy and the white spot syndromes (AZOOR complex) specific autoimmune diseases? Am J Ophthalmol 2003;135:380–381

8. Gass JDM. Acute posterior multifocal placoid pigment epitheliopathy. Arch Ophthalmol 1968;80:177–185

9. Grossniklaus HE, Gass JD. Clinicopathologic correlations of surgically excised type 1 and type 2 submacular choroidal neovascular membranes. Am J Ophthalmol 1998;126:59–69

10. Haen SP, Spaide RF. Fundus autofluorescence in multifocal choroiditis and panuveitis (in preparation)

11. Hegedus ZL. The probable involvement of soluble and deposited melanins, their intermediates and the reactive oxygen side-products in human diseases and aging. Toxicology 2000;145:85–101

12. Howe LJ, Woon H, Graham EM, Fitzke F, Bhandari A, Marshall J. Choroidal hypoperfusion in acute posterior multifocal placoid pigment epitheliopathy. An indocyanine green angiography study. Ophthalmology 1995;102:790–798

13. Jampol LM, Becker KG. White spot syndromes of the retina: a hypothesis based on the common genetic hypothesis of autoimmune/inflammatory disease. Am J Ophthalmol 2003;135:376–379

14. Kayatz P, Thumann G, Luther TT, Jordan JF, Bartz-Schmidt KU, Esser PJ, Schraermeyer U. Oxidation causes melanin fluorescence. Invest Ophthalmol Vis Sci 2001;42:241–246

15. Lofoco G, Ciucci F, Bardocci A, et al. Optical coherence tomography findings in a case of acute multifocal posterior placoid pigment epitheliopathy (AMPPPE). Eur J Ophthalmol. 2005;15:143–147

16. Matsumoto Y, Spaide RF. Autofluorescence imaging of acute syphilitic posterior placoid chorioretinitis. Retina (in press)

17. Nozik RA, Dorsch W. A new chorioretinopathy associated with anterior uveitis. Am J Ophthalmol 1973;76:758–762

18. Peters S, Kayatz P, Heimann K, Schraermeyer U. Subretinal injection of rod outer segments leads to an increase in the number of early-stage melanosomes in retinal pigment epithelial cells. Ophthalmic Res 2000;32:52–56

19. Rothova A, Berendschot TT, Probst K, et al. Birdshot chorioretinopathy: long-term manifestations and visual prognosis. Ophthalmology 2004;111:954–959

20. Ryan SJ, Maumenee AE. Birdshot retinochoroidopathy. Am J Ophthalmol 1980;89:31–45

21. Sarna T, Burke JM, Korytowski W, et al. Loss of melanin from human RPE with aging: possible role of melanin photooxidation. Exp Eye Res 2003;76:89–98

22. Schraermeyer U, Peters S, Thumann G, Kociok N, Heimann K. Melanin granules of retinal pigment epithelium are connected with the lysosomal degradation pathway. Exp Eye Res 1999;68:237–245

23. Schraermeyer U. The intracellular origin of the melanosome in pigment cells: a review of ultrastructural data. Histol Histopathol 1996;11:445–462

24. Slakter JS, Giovannini A, Yannuzzi LA,et al. Indocyanine green angiography of multifocal choroiditis. Ophthalmology 1997;104:1813–1819

25. Smith RE, Ganley JP, Knox DL. Presumed ocular histoplasmosis. II. Patterns of peripheral and peripapillary scarring in persons with nonmacular disease. Arch Ophthalmol 1972;87:251–257

26. Spaide RF, Klancnik JM Jr. Fundus autofluorescence and central serous chorioretinopathy. Ophthalmology 2005;112:825–833

27. Spaide RF, Noble K, Morgan A, Freund KB. Vitelliform macular dystrophy. Ophthalmology 2006;113:1392–1400

28. Spaide RF, Yannuzzi LA, Slakter J. Choroidal vasculitis in acute posterior multifocal placoid pigment epitheliopathy. Br J Ophthalmol 1991;75:685–7. Erratum in Br J Ophthalmol 1992;76:128

29. Spaide RF. Autofluorescence imaging of acute posterior multifocal placoid pigment epitheliopathy. Retina. 2006;26:479–842

30. Spaide RF. Collateral damage in acute zonal occult outer retinopathy. Am J Ophthalmol 2004;138:887–889

31. Spaide RF. Fundus autofluorescence and age-related macular degeneration. Ophthalmology 2003;110:392–399

32. Takagi T, Tsuda N, Watanabe F, Noguchi S. Subretinal precipitates of retinal detachments associated with intraocular tumors. Ophthalmologica 1988;197:120–126

33. Thumann G, Bartz-Schmidt KU, Kociok N, Heimann K, Schraemeyer U. Ultimate fate of rod outer segments in the retinal pigment epithelium. Pigment Cell Res 1999;12:311–315

34. Tran THA, Cassoux N, Bodaghi B, et al. Syphilitic uveitis in patients infected with human immunodeficiency virus. Graefes Arch Clin Exp Ophthalmol 2005;243:863–869

35. Bryan RG, Freund KB, Yannuzzi LA, et al. Multiple evanescent white dot syndrome in patients with multifocal choroiditis. Retina 2002;22:317–322

36. Gass JD, Hamed LM. Acute macular neuroretinopathy and multiple evanescent white dot syndrome occurring in the same patients. Arch Ophthalmol 1989;107:189–193

Fig. 16.1 a The normal retinal pigment epithelium (RPE) monolayer has a corresponding amount of autofluorescence (**b**). Inflammatory lesions have an alteration in color (**c**) and are often hyperautofluorescent in the acute phase (**d**). *e, f, g, h, see next page*

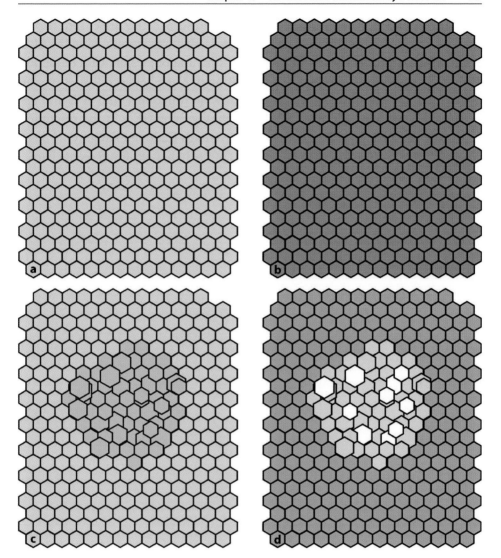

Fig. 16.1 *(Continued)* This increase in autofluorescence may arise from hypertrophy or hyperplasia of the RPE cells or increased fluorophores within the RPE. **e** Later there appears to be shrinkage of the inflammatory lesion, with retraction of the outer aspect of the lesion and formation of a gap between the lesion and the normal RPE monolayer. The gap contains no functional RPE cells and appears as a black band on autofluorescent photography (**f**). **g** In the resolution phase, the darker pigmented regions seen in image **e** adopt a flat greyish-black color. Along with the change in color, a loss of the hyperautofluorescent character occurs as well (**h**)

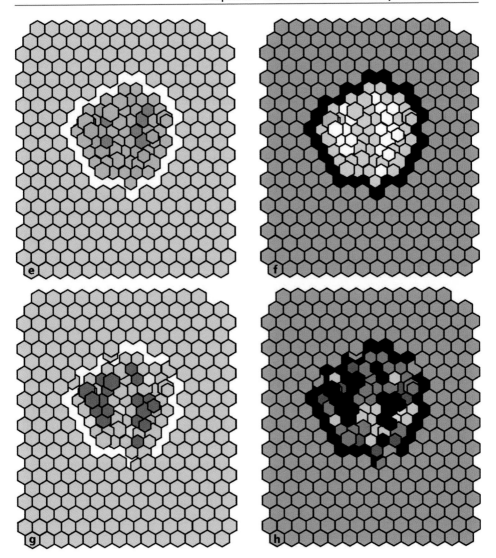

Fig. 16.2 a Color fundus photograph of the right eye shows multiple yellow-white placoid lesions in a patient with acute posterior placoid pigment epitheliopathy. **b** In the early phase of the fluorescein angiogram, there were many more areas of decreased fluorescence than the number of placoid lesions seen in the color photograph. **c** The late-phase fluorescein shows staining of some of the lesions (*arrow*), bordered by an adjacent blocking defect (*arrowhead*). **d** The autofluorescence photograph shows a band of hyperautofluorescence (*arrowhead*) corresponding to the blocking defect in image **c**. The area of hypoautofluorescence (*arrow*) corresponded to the area of staining during the fluorescein angiographic evaluation. (From Spaide RF. Autofluorescence imaging of acute posterior multifocal placoid pigment epitheliopathy. Retina 2006;26:479–482)

Fig. 16.3 a The same patient shown in Fig. 16.2, 2 weeks after presentation. The patient had an increase in both the size and number of visible lesions. In addition, many more of the lesions showed late fluorescein angiographic alterations. Note that the areas of hyperfluorescence (*arrows*) in the fluorescein angiogram (**a**) correspond to hypoautofluorescent regions in the autofluorescence photograph (*arrows*). The areas of blocking in the fluorescein angiogram (*arrowheads*) correspond to areas of hyperautofluorescence in the autofluorescence photograph

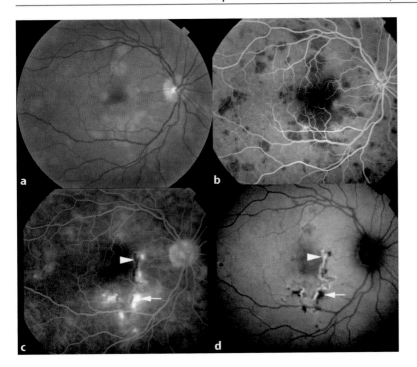

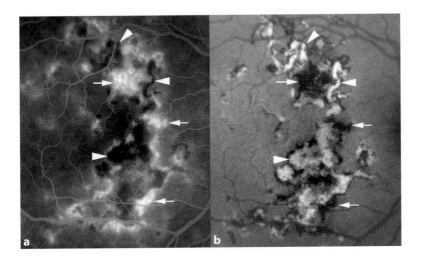

Fig. 16.4 a Color fundus photograph 4 weeks after presentation, showing healing of the lesions with increased pigmentation centrally (*arrowheads*) and decreased pigmentation (*arrows*). Note the decreased pigmentation forming haloes around the pigmented areas. **b** The autofluorescence photograph shows that the areas of pigmentation were hyperautofluorescent and the depigmented haloes were hypoautofluorescent. **c** Color photograph 6 months after presentation showing alteration in the pigment as seen in image **a**. Note that some of the pigmentation nearly disappeared, while other areas showed some decrease and other areas consolidated and became more flat-black. **d** The formerly hyperautofluorescent areas have become hypoautofluorescent. Note that the gap of hypoautofluorescence seen initially has tiny dots of autofluorescence, which may indicate repopulation of the atrophic areas

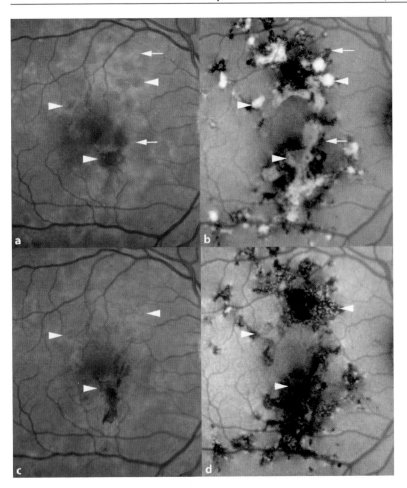

Fig. 16.5 a Color fundus photograph of the left eye showing yellow-white discoloration in the macular area extending from the optic nerve temporal to the fovea in a patient with acute syphilitic posterior placoid chorioretinitis. There is accumulation of yellowish material superotemporal to the fovea (*arrowheads*). **b** In the early-phase fluorescein angiogram, there was early blockage in the area of the yellowish material and at the temporal margin of the lesion. **c** In the late-phase fluorescein angiogram, there was staining of the lesion and optic nerve head. **d** The autofluorescence photograph shows hyperautofluorescence of the yellow clumps of material (*arrowheads* correspond to those in image **a** and a generalized increase in autofluorescence of the lesion. Small hypoautofluorescent points can be seen (*arrows in inset*). (From Matsumoto Y, Spaide RF. Autofluorescence imaging of acute syphilitic posterior placoid chorioretinitis. Retina, in press)

Fig. 16.6 a Follow-up of patient illustrated in Fig. 16.5, 4 months after treatment. Color fundus photograph of the left eye shows granularity of the pigmentation at the level of the retinal pigment epithelium and yellowish accumulation of material mimicking the material seen in Fig. 16.1a. **b** The red-free image shows the accumulated subretinal material. **c** Fluorescein angiogram shows a transmission defect in the region of the previous placoid change with small areas of blockage secondary to the subretinal yellowish material. **d** Autofluorescence photography shows that the yellowish material was hyperautofluorescent, the borders of which are more distinct than in the past

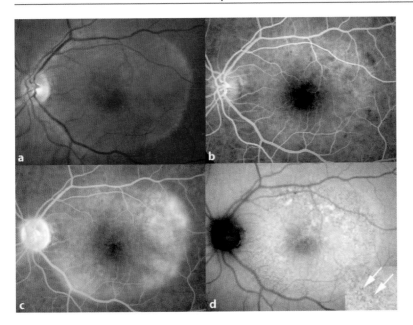

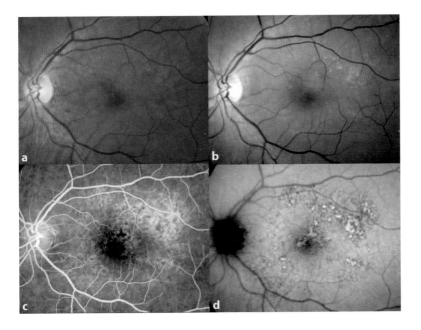

Fig. 16.7 a Color fundus photograph of the right eye showing a yellow-white placoid lesion that was more yellow and opaque at the outer borders in the macula, particularly superonasal to the fovea in this patient with acute syphilitic posterior placoid chorioretinitis. There were no yellow clumps of material, but there appeared to be atrophy or depigmentation at the level of the retinal pigment epithelium inferior to the fovea. **b** In the early phases of the fluorescein angiogram there was a slight transmission defect inferior to the fovea. **c** In the late phase of the fluorescein angiogram there was staining of the placoid lesion, particularly superonasal to the fovea, as well as staining of the optic nerve head. **d** The autofluorescence photograph demonstrates a hyperautofluorescence corresponding with the yellow-white placoid discoloration in the macula. Hypoautofluorescent dots are present inferior to the fovea in the region of the transmission defect (From Matsumoto Y, Spaide RF. Autofluorescence imaging of acute syphilitic posterior placoid chorioretinitis. Retina, in press)

Fig. 16.8 a Follow-up of patient illustrated in Fig. 16.7, 2 months after treatment. Color fundus photograph of the right eye shows some persistent depigmentation inferior to the fovea. **b,c** The fluorescein angiogram shows mild staining of the disc and a transmission defect in the inferior macular area in the right eye. **d** Autofluorescence photography shows nearly complete resolution of the hyperautofluorescence with no change in the hypoautofluorescent dots

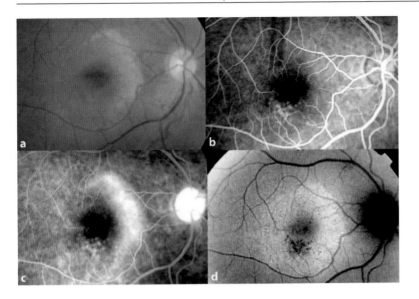

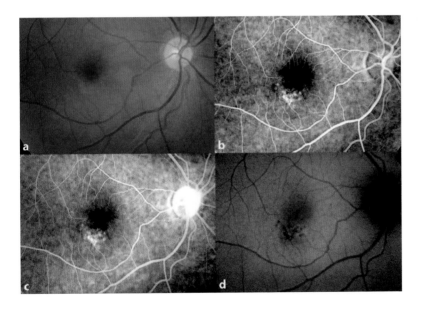

Fig. 16.9 a,b Color fundus photographs showing an asymmetrical presentation of multifocal choroiditis and panuveitis. The left eye has numerous chorioretinal scars and choroidal neovascularization. **c,d** The fluorescein angiogram shows subtle window defects in the right eye and larger scars in the left. The left eye has an area of choroidal neovascularization. Note the subtle blocking around the border of the choroidal neovascularization, probably secondary to enveloping hyperplastic retinal pigment epithelium seen in profile. **e,f** The indocyanine green angiogram shows some choroidal involvement in the left eye but does not show any involvement of the right eye. The choroidal neovascularization is poorly imaged in the left eye. **g,h** Autofluorescence photography shows innumerable hypoautofluorescent spots in the right eye. The left eye has both large and small hypoautofluorescent spots. Note that the outer border of the choroidal neovascularization (corresponding to the hypofluorescent boundary seen in image **d** is hyperautofluorescent

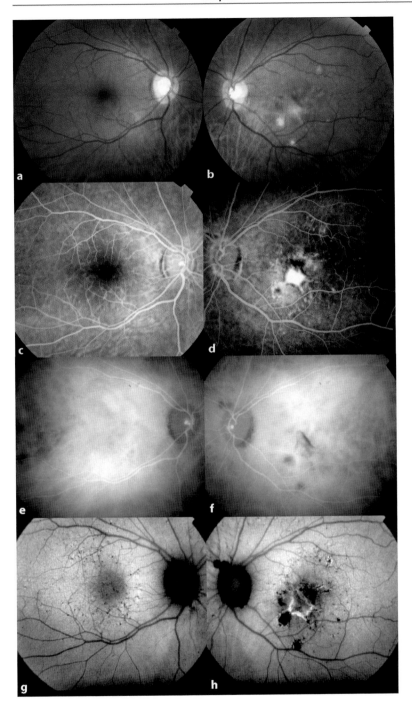

16.10 **a,b** The color fundus photograph of this 52-year-old patient with multifocal choroiditis shows bilateral chorioretinal scars and bilateral choroidal neovascularization. The patient was on systemic mycophenolate mofetil, tacrolimus, and prednisone. He had an old area of choroidal neovascularization in the left eye. In the right eye he had a more recent onset of choroidal neovascularization and was aggressively treated with intravitreal triamcinolone and bevacizumab. **c,d** The fluorescein angiogram of the right eye shows regressed choroidal neovascularization with no leakage. The left eye has a large area of choroidal neovascularization associated with retinal vascular and optic disc leakage. **e** Autofluorescence photography of the right eye shows several hypoautofluorescent spots and several contiguous areas of choroidal neovascularization. **f** There is a large neovascular lesion in the left eye highlighted by hyperautofluorescence. Note the small ringlike areas of hyperautofluorescence nasal to the disc, probably indicative of small foci of choroidal neovascularization (From Haen SP, Spaide RF. Fundus autofluorescence in multifocal choroiditis and panuveitis. In preparation)

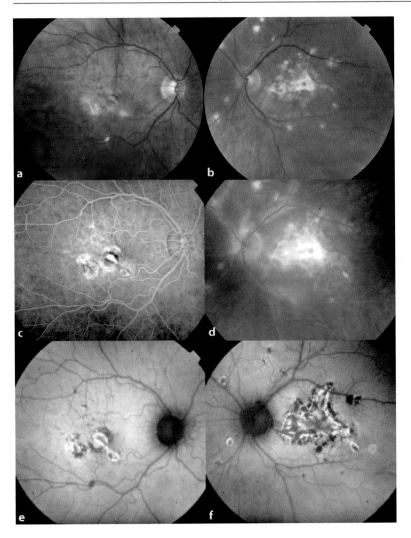

Fig. 16.11 **a** Color photograph of the right involved fundus showing yellowish drusen-like material at the outer border of the lesion in a patient with acute zonal occult outer retinopathy. **b** Fluorescein angiography shows a transmission defect in the central portion of the lesion and blocking where the yellowish material accumulated (*arrows*). The indocyanine green angiogram in the early (**c**) and middle phases (**d**) of the sequence shows hypofluorescence within the lesion (*arrows*) without diminution of the fluorescence of the underlying larger choroidal vessels, suggesting the presence of choriocapillaris atrophy (From Spaide RF. Collateral damage in acute zonal occult outer retinopathy. Am J Ophthalmol. 2004;138:887–889)

Fig. 16.12 Autofluorescence photograph of acute zonal occult outer retinopathy. The autofluorescence photograph shows intense hyperautofluorescence at the outer border of the lesion corresponding to the yellowish drusen-like material, consistent with the accumulation of large amounts of lipofuscin. The central portions of the lesion were hypoautofluorescent, consistent with atrophy of the retinal pigment epithelium

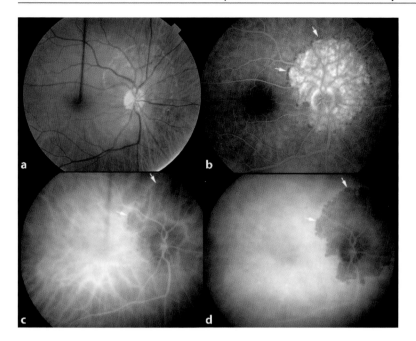

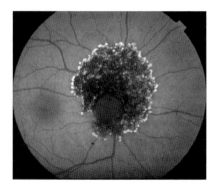

Fig. 16.13 Same patient as shown in Figs. 16.11 and 16.12, but 2.5 years later. **a** Note the decrease in prominence of the outer border of the lesion. **b** The outer border of the lesion shows less prominent hyperautofluorescence, but the inner portions of the lesion show more profound atrophy

Fig. 16.14 This patient had widespread involvement with acute zonal occult outer retinopathy. Note that the exaggerated findings in the photograph mirror those seen in Fig. 16.12 *(Courtesy of Lawrence Yannuzzi, MD)*

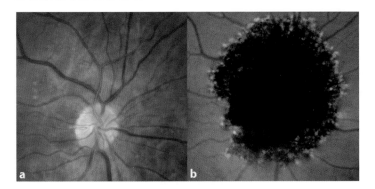

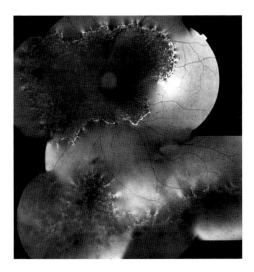

Fig. 16.15 **a** This 29-year-old woman presented with an enlarged blind spot during visual field testing, as well as small white dots. **b** Indocyanine green angiography revealed multiple hypofluorescent dots. A diagnosis of multiple evanescent white dot syndrome was made. **c** An autofluorescence photograph taken at the time shows no spots but does show a subtle increase in autofluorescence in a zone around the nerve. **d** When examined 6 days later, the spots were not present. **e** The patient had an increasing visual field deficit and photopsias. When examined 2 years later, she was seen to have an alteration of the color of the retinal pigment epithelium (*arrowheads*). **f** Autofluorescence photography showed a large region of decreased and mottled autofluorescence surrounding the nerve. A diagnosis of acute zonal occult outer retinopathy was made

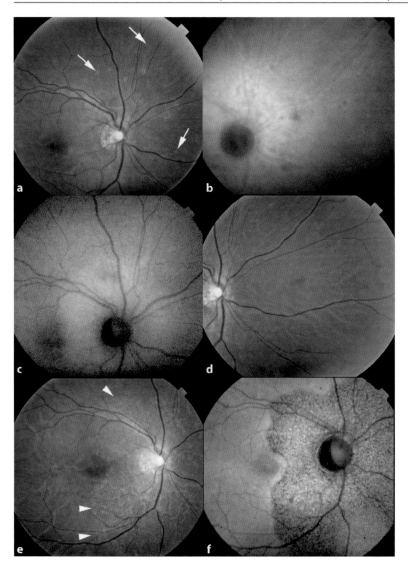

Fig. 16.16 a Color photograph of a patient with birdshot chorioretinopathy. **b** The comparative autofluorescent photograph. Note that depigmented areas within the choroid in the color photograph do not necessarily correspond to areas of retinal pigment epithelium damage in the autofluorescence photograph

Fig. 16.17 a An end-stage case of birdshot chorioretinopathy shows optic atrophy, sheathing of the retinal vessels, and widespread pigmentary disturbance. **b** Montage autofluorescence photograph centered on the optic nerve shows extensive damage to the retinal pigment epithelium

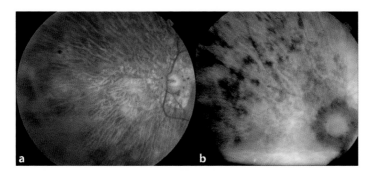

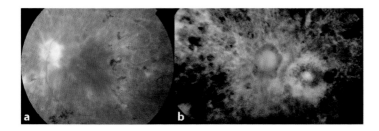

Autofluorescence from the Outer Retina and Subretinal Space

Richard F. Spaide

17.1
Introduction

Most diseases causing increased autofluorescence do so because of a corresponding increase in fluorophores in the retinal pigment epithelium (RPE). This chapter covers diseases and conditions causing increased autofluorescence generated from the outer retina and subretinal space in addition to the autofluorescence normally originating from the RPE (Fig. 17.1). This autofluorescence arising from the retina and subretinal space generally does not come from lipofuscin as such, because lipofuscin is a mixture of material found in an intracellular organelle, the lysosome. These diseases are generally associated with physical separation of the outer segments from the RPE, thus hindering normal phagocytosis of the shed outer segments of the photoreceptors. The shed photoreceptor outer segments are theorized to accumulate on the outer retina and in the subretinal space [1, 2].

The teleological argument for rapid photoreceptor outer segment shedding is for the removal of cellular material damaged during normal use. The outer segments contain retinoids, molecules utilized because of their ability to absorb and utilize light. These molecules are capable of reacting with normal constituents of the outer segments to produce novel molecules. The outer segments also contain proteins and large proportions of highly polyunsaturated fatty acids, all of which are susceptible to oxidative damage [3–5]. Accumulation of shed outer segments allows the amassing of the damaged materials destined to be removed by normal outer segment turnover and renewal. The buildup of these damaged molecules not only confers increased fluorescence but also has the potential to eventually load the RPE cells with an abundance of potentially toxic compounds once cleared by phagocytosis. A large number of fluorophores can be detected in lipofuscin, and the bulk of them originate in the retina. Rats lacking photoreceptor s due to genetic defects or those unable to phagocytose outer segments show markedly reduced lipofuscin formation within the RPE [6, 7] (see chapter 1). Although reactions in the outer segments involving retinoids may not be the sole means of fluorophore development, the mechanism of formation of these fluorophores [8] may serve as a model for the occurrence of autofluorescence in the outer retina and subretinal space.

Light sensitivity of the retinal photoreceptors is conferred by visual pigments derived from vitamin A. The light-sensitive portion, 11-*cis*-retinal, is bound to the transmembrane portion of the photoreceptor cell opsin. On absorption of a photon, 11-*cis*-retinal is isomerized to all-*trans*-retinal (ATR), and the conformational change in the opsin leads to activation of G-proteins and a cascade of signaling reactions to cause an electrical response in the photoreceptor. To be useful in future phototransduction reactions, the ATR needs to be converted back into the 11-cis conformation. The first step is conversion of the all-*trans*-retinal to all-*trans*-retinol by all-*trans*-retinol-dehydrogenase. Most ATR enters this reaction, but some ATR, existing in a free state not bound to an opsin, can enter into a nonenzymatic reaction with phosphatidylethanolamine (PE) to create N-retinylidene-PE. Reaction with a second ATR creates a bisretinoid molecule A2-PE-H_2, which appears to undergo spontaneous oxidation to form A2-PE, a molecule named to reflect the molar presence of two retinal molecules derived from vitamin A and the phosphatidylethanolamine. A2-PE-H_2, A2-PE, and A2E are all fluorescent, with the peak wavelength being the longest for A2-PE-H_2 and shortest for A2E [9].

Additional products ultimately derived from ATR have been described. These include all-*trans*-retinal dimmers (atRAL) that can react with PE [10]. The resultant molecule, atRAL dimmer-PE, along with atRAL also have a fluorescence spectra that is red-shifted compared with A2E. These molecules form in the retina prior to phagocytosis by the RPE and lead to increased A2E within the RPE cells. Once phagocytosed by the RPE cell, the abnormally cross-linked retinoids and the oxidized protein and lipid moieties mutually contribute in a synergistic fashion to lipofuscinogenesis through intersecting pathways (see Chap. 1) [5, 11–14].

17.2
Animal Models

Many of the diseases have no direct animal model. However, the Royal College of Surgeons (RCS) rat develops a dystrophy caused by the inability of RPE cells to phagocytose outer segments [15]. These animals develop a deposition of shed, but not phagocytosed, outer segments in the subretinal space that remain attached to the retina if the retina and RPE are physically separated. Ultrastructural examination of this material has shown degenerated photoreceptor cells and outer segments. This material is highly autofluorescent and when evaluated by thin-layer chromatography was found to contain several fluorophores [7]. Several fluorophores emitting red, yellow, and yellow-green light were found in normal rats. Three additional fluorophores, all emitting intense orange fluorescence under ultraviolet excitation, were either not found or were only faintly visible in normal rats [7]. One constituent fluorophore was determined to be A2-PE in later analysis [16, 17]. Gene transfer of Mertk, the defective gene encoding a receptor tyrosine kinase in RCS rats through a replication-deficient adenovirus vector, corrected the RPE phagocytosis defect [18]. The rats having viral gene replacement therapy did not develop the accumulation of degenerated outer segment material in the subretinal space, but they did have phagosomes containing lamellated packets of disk membranes that were fluorescent.

Animal models generated to study adenosine binding cassette protein A4 (ABCA4) mutations supply additional information [16]. ABCA4 mutations lie at the heart of Stargardt disease [19]. ABCA4 is a member of a large superfamily of transmembrane transport proteins that use adenosine triphosphate (ATP) to translocate molecules across cell membranes. ABCA4 is located along the rims and incisures of the outer segment disks and appears to be involved in the transport of N-retinylidene-PE. Mutation of the gene results in a protein with decreased or absent transport abilities. Retinal tissue from abc4a-/- mice showed elevated levels of atRAL, N-retinylidene-PE, and A2-PE [9]. It seems likely that the improper transport of the N-retinylidene-PE from the lumen to the cytoplasmic side of the disk membrane leads to the formation of ATR derivatives within the outer segment prior to phagocytosis. Although this exact mechanism is not implicated in the diseases highlighted in this chapter (see chapter 9), the pathophysiologic mechanism has germane elements. Improper transport of retinoids may hinder their correct metabolism, with the production of undesirable derivatives instead. These derivatives are autofluorescent and potentially toxic.

17.3
Histopathology

Published histopathologic material on diseases is notably absent for many diseases in this classification. Histopathologic photographs from a case of de Venecia of acute central serous chorioretinopathy following high-dose corticosteroids given for renal failure complicated by aspergillosis infection of the optic nerve and orbital apex was published anecdotally by Gass in his atlas [20]. The patient had no light perception, and the enucleated eye showed extensive subretinal fibrinous exudation. This case was enucleated prior to the time increased autofluorescence is usually seen in cases of central serous chorioretinopathy, and the severity of the patient findings and concurrent medical problems were not characteristic for a routine patient with typical central serous chorioretinopathy.

Histopathologic examination of vitelliform macular dystrophy (VMD) has been performed for patients who were well past the egg-yolk stage. O'Gorman et al. examined the donor eyes from a 69-year-old with VMD. The RPE cells had large amounts of lipofuscin, and there was an accumulation of heterogeneous material located between the RPE and Bruch's membrane [21]. There was foveal photoreceptor loss, and the subretinal space contained collections of outer segment debris and phagocytic cells. Fragieh et al. [22] reported the findings of an 80-year-old who had a family history of VMD but did not have documented accumulations of vitelliform material. There were flattened RPE cells containing an abnormal amount of lipofuscin. The patient had a PAS-positive, acid-mucopolysaccharide-negative, electron-dense accumulation of finely granular material in the subretinal space. Weingeist and associates reported a case of VMD in a 28-year-old with a scrambled-egg lesion [23]. The patient had RPE abnormalities with an abnormal accumulation of lipopigment within RPE cells and macrophages in the subretinal space and within the choroid.

Arnold and colleagues [24] reported the histopathologic findings of four eyes with adult-onset foveomacular vitelliform dystrophy (AFVD) and retrospectively found 10 additional eyes. They found collections of extracellular material in the subretinal space. The bulk of the debris consisted of rounded or elongated densely packed multilamellar bodies that appeared to be derived from the breakdown of outer segment discs. The retina anterior to the subretinal material showed attenuation of the photoreceptors, especially in the central fovea. The subretinal material was bounded posteriorly by the RPE, which was attenuated centrally. At the edge of the lesion, the RPE was hypertrophic, heaped up at the edge of the lesion with reduplication of the RPE monolayer. Some of the RPE cells were disrupted and appeared to be disgorging their contents into the subretinal space. The authors attributed the yellow color to lipofuscin in the subretinal space. Additional cases of AFVD have been reported, but almost all were confined to eyes in which the yellow material had gone away, except for a report by Dubovy and associates. They found lipofuscin-laden macrophages in the subretinal space and also lipofuscin in the underlying RPE. They attributed the yellow color to the presence of lipofuscin-containing cells in the subretinal space [25]. Eckardt and colleagues performed a macular translocation on a patient with AFVD and surgically removed the vitelliform lesion en bloc [26]. They noticed that the yellow vitelliform material dissolved away during processing, leaving the RPE behind. This raises the possibility that other studies reporting the histopathology of vitelliform lesions may have had similar dissolution of the vitelliform material during processing.

Shields and associates examined choroidal nevi, hemangiomas, and melanomas with overlying orange pigment and found that the pigment corresponded to lipofuscin in macrophages in the subretinal space [27]. Takagi and colleagues found that the retinal detachments associated with intraocular tumors contained subretinal precipitates that were actually foam cells located around degenerated outer and inner segments of photoreceptor cells [28]. These foam cells contained lipid droplets, lysosomes with lipofuscin and melanin.

17.4
Ocular Imaging

Autofluorescence photography shows increased autofluorescence originating from the posterior surface of the retina and subretinal space in the cases shown in Fig. 17.1. Associated with the increase in autofluorescence is an increase in the thickness of an accumulation of shaggy material on the posterior surface of the retina. If there is a large amount of accumulation there may be a gravitating amassing of similar material at the bottom edge of the associated detachment. The autofluorescence appears to be imaged more prominently by the wavelengths used with fundus camera autofluorescence photography than those used with the scanning laser ophthalmoscope.

There are two reasons that may explain this difference. First, the confocal nature of the imaging by scanning laser ophthalmoscopic approaches rejects fluorescence from planes that are not conjugate with those targeted. In cases where there is a neurosensory detachment and the focus is directed at the level of the RPE, the fluorescence from the retina may be rejected. Fundus cameras do not have the ability to reject light originating from adjacent layers.

The second reason involves the fluorophores involved. Scanning laser ophthalmoscopes use wavelengths selected to optimize the detection of lipofuscin. The fluorophores that accumulate in the retina, such as the precursors to A2E, fluoresce at longer wavelengths than do the end-products that accumulate as lipofuscin [9]. The barrier filter of the fundus camera has a longer wavelength pass-band than does the scanning laser ophthalmoscope, and the pass-band straddles the wavelengths produced by the precursor fluorophores. Because of the difference in wavelengths used, the light from the retina would account for a greater proportion of the total fundus fluorescence with a fundus camera than a scanning laser ophthalmoscope. Because this chapter examines autofluorescence originating from the outer retina and subretinal space, emphasis will be placed on studies done with fundus camera imaging in order to develop concepts that are applicable to any type of autofluorescence imaging.

Fundus autofluorescence dose not exist in isolation. An important utility of an imaging method lies in the integration of new information provided with alternate methods of imaging that may provide additional information. Autofluorescence photography supplies information about the physiology of a given disorder across the x, y plane and with stereo imaging, a limited amount in the z-axis. However stereo autofluorescence imaging is not routinely performed in modern workflows. On the other hand, optical coherence tomography (OCT) provides excellent anatomic information about the cross-section of the retina, and new spectral OCT machines provide three-dimensional images of the anatomy of the posterior pole (see Chap. 3.3). Additional imaging methods such as color photography and angiography can also be integrated into the imaging mix. The integrated information is the basis for patient evaluation.

17.5
Central Serous Chorioretinopathy

Central serous chorioretinopathy is a condition characterized by idiopathic leaks from the level of the RPE leading to serous retinal detachment. In the early phases of the disease, the visual acuity may be good despite the presence of the macular detachment, and after resolution the acuity often shows improvement. More chronic forms of central serous chorioretinopathy are associated with atrophic and degenerative changes of the retina and RPE and consequently with visual acuity decline [29]. In addition, subretinal deposits are seen, some being ascribed to lipid or proteins such as fibrin [29]. Older patients or those taking corticosteroids may develop a prominent accumulation of yellowish subretinal material. Our knowledge of central serous chorioretinopathy has been limited by the lack of significant amounts of histopathologic study of the disorder. Investigational tools such as fluorescein and indocyanine green angiography have provided some insight into the hemodynamics and fluid dynamics. OCT has provided additional clues about the size and elevation of detachments [30], the development of retinal atrophy, and the correlates to visual acuity in resolved central serous chorioretinopathy [31].

Patients with acute leaks imaged within the first month have minimal abnormalities seen in their autofluorescence photography, other than a slight increase in autofluorescence of the serous detachment (Fig. 17.2). Over the next months the area of detachment becomes increasingly hyperautofluorescent. This autofluorescence is diffuse, but it contains discrete granules as well. The subretinal hyperautofluorescent granules correspond to pinpoint subretinal precipitates (Fig. 17.3). The hyperautofluorescence is generally uniformly distributed, but the material often gravitates inferiorly or collects in deposits at the border of the detachment (Figs. 17.2 and 17.3). The subretinal material blocks the background fluorescence during fluorescein angiography, particularly where the material aggregated or settled. Pronounced accumulation of material produces the appearance of yellow flecks in some patients (Fig. 17.4). OCT has demonstrated that areas with increased autofluorescence had an accumulation of material on the outer surface of the retina that was proportional in thickness with the amount of autofluorescence seen. Indeed, central serous chorioretinopathy detachments can look frankly yellow over time (Figs. 17.5 and 17.6). Because of the way a fundus camera images the fundus, the observed autofluorescence is a summation of the autofluorescence from the retina and underlying RPE. Patients with decreased autofluorescence have little accumulation of material on the outer retina, but they also have attenuation of the reflected signal from the RPE, with increased visibility of the underlying choroid by OCT suggesting the presence of retinal pigment epithelial atrophy (Fig. 17.7). A few granules of material can be seen on the surface of the retinal pigment epithelium in some patients. Patients with chronic disease have varying degrees of atrophy, including broader areas of geographic atrophy in the macula and within fluid tracts descending inferiorly. Descending tracts of more recent origin and the outer borders of more chronic descending tracts (Fig. 17.8) are hyperautofluorescent. Autofluorescence imaging soon after the development of central serous chorioretinopathy shows little or no change in the autofluorescence pattern in the area around the leak, although the leak site may be somewhat hypoautofluorescent. Patients with more chronic leaks can have decreased autofluorescence surrounding the known leaks. This area of hypoautofluorescence appears to expand in size with increasing chronicity of the leak. Patients known to have a history of chronic central serous chorioretinopathy that had been inactive for several years are left with hypoautofluorescent areas and no hyperautofluorescent regions.

In experimental retinal detachment there is abnormal production [32], assembly [33, 34], and shedding [35] of the outer segments owing to the lack of direct apposition and phagocytosis by the RPE. In rhegmatogenous retinal detachments, the outer segments are washed out of the subretinal space by flow induced by ocular saccades and convection currents. Deposition of the outer segments in the trabecular meshwork can lead to decreased outflow and increased intraocular pressure, as seen in the Schwartz-Matsuo phenomenon [36]. In central serous retinopathy there is a loculated fluid space with no means of escape for the shed photoreceptor outer segments (Fig. 17.9). Accumulation of the photoreceptor outer segments, admixed with possible lipoproteins from the serous fluid leaking into the subretinal space, may lead to the buildup of the autofluorescent material seen in these patients. Accumulation of this material may explain previously reported findings of yellow material accumulating in the subretinal space in patients with central serous chorioretinopathy [37, 38]. The small punctuate areas of hyperautofluorescence are colocalized with the small white dots seen by ophthalmoscopy on the undersurface of the retina. The number of the dots can vary in number, but there is not much variability in size of the dots. The uniformity of size and their autofluorescent nature suggest that these dots may be macrophages, engorged with phagocytosed outer segments. Macrophages containing outer segments have been seen in the subretinal space during histopathologic examination of retinoblastoma and choroidal melanoma [28].

Atrophy of the RPE and the decreasing amount of material on the outer surface of the retina has been seen in the same patients, suggesting that atrophy of both occurs in parallel. In rhegmatogenous retinal detachment, changes occur both in the retina and RPE [32]. Patients with central serous chorioretinopathy retain fairly good levels of visual acuity, suggesting that the perturbations induced by the shallow circumscribed retinal detachment are less acutely severe than those caused by rhegmatogenous retinal detachment, but the chronicity of central serous chorioretinopathy may promote the accumulation of material in the subretinal space. Patients with a history of central serous chorioretinopathy with resolution of subretinal fluid have been seen to have a lack of hyperautofluorescence, suggesting that the hyperautofluorescent material could be cleared with time.

Additional deposition of material, including subretinal lipid and fibrin, has been described in patients with central serous chorioretinopathy. Subretinal lipid is a term used to refer to aggregates of spheroidal, yellowish, hard-edged granules similar to those seen in diabetic retinopathy or choroidal neovascularization (CNV). The "lipid" is thought to be composed of precipitated lipoproteins. Lipid deposits are not autofluorescent. Subretinal "fibrin" is a greyish-white feathery-edged placoid deposition of what appears to be protein, and may in fact be fibrin. Subretinal fibrin is not autofluorescent.

17.6
Adult-Onset Foveomacular Vitelliform Dystrophy

Adult-onset foveomacular vitelliform dystrophy (AFVD), a pattern dystrophy affecting mid- to advanced-aged adults, is associated with the deposition of yellowish material in a region one-quarter to one disk diameter in size, and sometimes larger, under the macula. Many differing clinical pictures appear to be lumped together under this rubric. Some patients have what appears to be an irregular confluence of yellow flecks in the fovea; others have a multiradiate pattern with branching rays of material extending from central collection; others have a small area of yellowish material with a central pigmented dot; and some have a large vitelliform collection. The fluorescein pattern can vary among these different types of presentation, from central blocking with surrounding transmission defects to what appears to be frank leakage during fluorescein angiography (Fig. 17.10). The latter fluorescein angiographic appearance is usually associated with larger vitelliform collections. Some patients have had a leak similar to that seen in central serous chorioretinopathy visible during fluorescein angiography and later developed findings identical to AFVD [38]. It is possible that AFVD is more than one entity that causes the collection of yellowish subretinal material in an adult patient. For patients with leakage, it may be possible that separation of the retina from the RPE hinders normal outer-segment phagocytosis and turnover, allowing accumulation of subretinal material. This may not be true for all forms of what is called AFVD, however.

17.7
Choroidal Tumors

Choroidal hemangiomas may be circumscribed or diffuse. The circumscribed hemangiomas are orange-red tumefactions that often have associated subretinal fluid and yellowish subretinal material over the tumefaction (Fig. 17.11). Fluorescein angiography shows an early filling of large vascular channels within the tumefaction, leakage from the tumefaction, blockage of the underlying fluorescence by the yellow material, and varying degrees of secondary retinal changes from chronic detachment. The yellow pigment is highly autofluorescent. Descending tracts such as those seen in central serous chorioretinopathy have been documented in patients with choroidal hemangiomas [39]. Choroidal nevi and melanomas are also associated with orange subretinal material that is autofluorescent (Fig. 17.12). Histopathologic evaluation of these cases has shown the material to be lipofuscin contained within macrophages in the subretinal space. Given the finding that the vitelliform material in AFVD dissolved during processing, there remains the possibility that extracellular material could have been washed away as well in cases of choroidal tumors. Histopathologic examination of retinoblastoma cases has shown macrophages in the subretinal space containing lipofuscin [28]. It is possible that the color of the deposited material varies with the associated disease. The macrophages in the subretinal space in cases of melanoma also have a large number of melanin granules, which may account for the pigment's looking orange in melanomas and nevi but yellow in hemangiomas.

17.8
Cystoid Macular Edema

Severe cystoid macular edema is associated with serous detachment of the macula as seen by OCT. Prior to widespread use of OCT, the presence of serous detachments was not mentioned in detailed reviews of the disorder, even by Gass. Patients with serous retinal detachment of the macula may develop an accumulation of material on the outer surface of the retina that has a subtle yellow color. (Gass noted yellow deposits in patients with cystoid macular edema without commenting on their origin.) Autofluorescence photography shows a slight hyperautofluorescence of the yellow subretinal material (Fig. 17.13).

17.9
Choroidal Neovascularization

Choroidal neovascularization (CNV) is commonly associated with intraretinal or subretinal yellowish material referred to as lipid. Close examination of the lipid can reveal more than one phenotype of the yellowish material. The true "lipid" is probably a lipoprotein of vascular origin (Figs. 17.14 and 17.15). Patients with CNV can have larger globular collections of yellowish subretinal material as well. These globular areas occur in regions of neurosensory detachment. Typical lipid is not autofluorescent and may be slightly hypoautofluorescent, whereas the globular areas are hyperautofluorescent.

17.10
Optic Pit Maculopathy

Serous macular detachment eventually occurs in 40–50% of patients with optic nerve pits [40]. Although serous macular detachment is the most common sequela leading to vision loss in these patients, the origin of the fluid remains to be elucidated. Various theories have implicated fluid entry from either the vitreous cavity or from cerebrospinal fluid via the peripapillary subarachnoid space [41, 42]. In any case, the subretinal fluid causes a disruption of the normal retinal anatomy, resulting in a lack of apposition between photoreceptor outer segments and RPE. Interestingly patients with serous detachment of the macula secondary to an optic nerve pit develop yellow subretinal flecks (Figs. 17.16–17.18). These accretions are intensely autofluorescent and are solely limited to areas of serous retinal detachment. The serous detachment separates the photoreceptor outer segments from the underlying RPE and potentially inhibits proper phagocytosis of shed outer segments. Accumulation of the shed outer segments would allow accrual of fluorophores under the outer retinal surface. After surgery, flattening of the detachment is met with resorption of the yellow material.

An alternate explanation for the formation of the subretinal precipitates is that they represent depositions of fibrin or lipoprotein. The deposition of subretinal fibrin in conjunction with neurosensory detachments has been well documented in central serous retinopathy [43]. Fibrin occurs as feathery-edged greyish white sheets overlying active leaks. There was no evidence of focal leaks from the RPE in patients with optic pit maculopathy. Lipoprotein accumulation is unlikely for a variety of reasons. First, the retinal detachment in optic nerve pit cases is not necessarily contiguous with the pit itself; there is often an intervening area of retinal schisis-like change. No increased autofluorescence is seen outside of the detachment. Second, there is no observable fluorescein leakage into the detachment in these cases, making any proposed source of the lipoprotein seem cryptic. Third, neither cerebrospinal fluid nor the vitreous, both proposed as the origin of the fluid in optic disk maculopathy, are commonly thought to contain significant amounts of lipoprotein. Fourth, the yellow precipitates normally attributed to lipoprotein, such as exudates seen in diabetic retinopathy or CNV, are not autofluorescent.

17.11
Tractional Detachment of the Macula

Vitreomacular traction syndrome places tensile forces on the macula and is associated with thickening and polycystic changes in the macula. Some cases of vitreomacular traction cause frank detachment of the central macula with no concomitant leak. A yellow discoloration develops if there is a gross elevation of the central macula, and sometimes a prominent amount of subretinal yellow material can accumulate (Figs. 17.19–17.21). These detachments have the same yellow dots that eyes with central serous chorioretinopathy have. This confirms the notion that the dots are not directly related to a leak but rather to the detachment. Over time, the dots change location but do not increase in size, suggesting that they may be lipofuscin-laden macrophages. Surgical removal of the traction is met with a slow resolution of the detachment and clearance of the yellow material. Focal traction on the central fovea can cause a localized detachment with accumulation of material on the outer surface of the foveola, creating a yellow spot that is hyperautofluorescent. Focal detachment of the foveola was hypothesized by Gass to be a stage in macular hole formation. While this supposition was found to occur in only a minority of cases of premacular hole states, Gass did remark on the yellow appearance of the detachment [44].

17.12
Persistent Subretinal Fluid after Retinal Reattachment Surgery

After all forms of retinal reattachment surgery, but particularly after scleral buckling procedures with extensive cryopexy, a shallow amount of subretinal fluid may remain for many months. In 1968 Machemer published a paper examining the effects of retinal reattachment in owl monkeys and noticed small collections of subretinal fluid in some of them [45]. Curiously, the blebs showed intense fluorescence with the filters used for fluorescein angiography prior to injection of the fluorescein. In retrospect, this finding was probably autofluorescence. In a paper published by Robertson in 1978 [46], delay in reabsorption of subretinal fluid was found to be associated with the accumulation of cream-colored aggregates on the posterior surface of the retina. When the subretinal fluid was analyzed, macrophages containing complex melanosomes, lipid particles, and membranous cytoplasmic bodies theorized to be derived from photoreceptors were found. Later study with OCT confirmed that the small blebs after retinal reattachment surgery contained serous fluid, that they could have a yellowish-orange color cast, and that some patients may have a shallow detachment of the fovea [47–49]. These patients often have improved visual acuity after the retinal reattachment surgery but complain bitterly about their central vision if there is a foveal detachment. OCT shows an accumulation of outer retinal material that is autofluorescent. With flattening of the localized detachment, a mound of yellow material often remains (Figs. 17.22 and 17.23).

17.13
Acute Exudative Polymorphous Vitelliform Maculopathy

Acute exudative polymorphous vitelliform maculopathy is an exceedingly rare disorder causing an exudative detachment of the retina with slow resorption of the subretinal fluid [50, 51]. Over weeks, an accumulation of yellowish material appears in multiple blebs except for in the central macula, where there appears to be a confluence of the blebs creating a collapse of the yellowish material into a gravitating fluid level. Eventually the yellow material disappears, and there is an incomplete recovery of visual acuity. Interestingly, the patients have abnormal electro-oculogram (EOG) light peak:dark trough ratios that do not change even though the visible manifestations improve, and the patients do not appear to have an abnormality in the bestrophin and peripherin/RDS genes [51, 52].

Although the exudative detachment would seem to set the stage for accumulation of nonphagocytosed outer segments in the subretinal space, the volume of accumulated material seems remarkable. Gass, who described the disorder, thought the material was not lipoproteins from the choroid. Consistent with this is the finding that the accumulated material is exceedingly hyperautofluorescent. Interestingly, a patient examined with fluorescein angiography showed a decrease in the background choroidal fluorescence somewhat similar to that seen in Stargardt disease. This suggests that the RPE in patients with acute exudative polymorphous vitelliform maculopathy may have excessive amounts of lipofuscin (Fig. 17.24).

Three patients have been described with findings very similar to acute exudative polymorphous vitelliform maculopathy except that the patients had melanomas [53]. The authors thought the patients' ocular manifestations were related to a paraneoplastic process. Exudation into the subretinal space has been reported with paraneoplastic processes such as bilateral uveomelanocytic proliferation, but the polymorphous vitelliform accumulation in these patients raises the possibility that RPE phagocytosis of the outer segments may have been altered by the paraneoplastic process. The finding of persistent depression of the abnormal EOG light peak: dark trough ratios with no bestrophin gene abnormalities suggests that the decreased ratios may be related to an undefined genetic abnormality or to an acquired disorder of RPE function. This abnormality of RPE function is a transient, nonrecurring event, implying that it is acquired. This defect appears to involve the RPE's ability to remove subretinal fluid, and possibly outer segments, from the subretinal space.

17.14
Vitelliform Macular Dystrophy

Vitelliform macular dystrophy type 2 (VMD2, also known as Best's disease) is an autosomal-dominant disease caused by mutation in the gene coding for bestrophin, a Ca^{2+}-sensitive Cl^- channel protein located on the basolateral membrane of retinal pigment epithelial cells [19, 54, 55]. VMD2 has a highly variable phenotypic expression but complete penetrance of abnormalities in the rise of light current as measured during an EOG, which is related to defective Cl^- conductance from the flawed bestrophin protein [54–56]. In affected individuals, VMD2 is characterized by the variable deposition of yellowish material, which in the past has been attributed to lipofuscin in the RPE (Figs. 17.25–17.31) [57–59].

The phenotypic appearance varies with the stage of the disease. An accumulation of yellow material in the central macula causes a circumscribed, dome-shaped lesion one or two disc diameters across that resembles an egg yolk (hence the descriptive name, vitelliform). (See Figs. 17.26 and 17.27.) There is a variable amount of admixed transparent fluid, the proportion of which seems to increase over time. Over years, the material in the subretinal space may gravitate inferiorly to produce a fluid level between the yellow substance and the transparent subretinal fluid seen in these patients (Fig. 17.28). Eventually the yellow material appears to dissipate, leaving isolated clumps of matter, often at the edges of the macular lesion. Autofluorescence imaging has shown that after disappearance of the central vitelliform lesion (Fig. 17.29) there can be widespread deposition of fluorophores throughout the fundus, often in striking fractal-like patterns of spokes and globular elements (Fig. 17.30) [60]. Additional insights were suggested after examining the autofluorescence and OCT findings in patients with central serous chorioretinopathy [2, 61]. These patients had OCT evidence of accumulating autofluorescent material on the outer surface of the retina in areas of retinal detachment, and this material became increasingly thick and autofluorescent with duration of the disease. This material, thought to be aggregates of shed photoreceptor outer segments, may accumulate in part because of the lack of apposition of the retina to the RPE, which decreased the phagocytosis of the outer segments within the loculated confines of the central serous chorioretinopathy detachment [2]. Also, several patients have been described who had focal central serous leaks and later developed yellowish accumulation of subretinal material mimicking that seen in AFVD and VMD2 [37, 38.] Although the basic defect in VMD is related to an abnormal Cl^- channel in the RPE and thus may differ from the underlying etiologic cause of central serous chorioretinopathy, the net result in VMD patients may be the presence of subretinal fluid and associated altered outer segment turnover as a consequence.

In VMD2 the size of the lesion is correlated with the patient's age. With increasing chronicity of the lesions, there is central clearing of the yellow material, but there is usually accumulation of yellow material at the outer borders of the lesion. During fluorescein angiography, patients almost always have some hyperfluorescence within the lesion except when there is blocking by thick areas of yellowish material. This hyperfluorescence has four main forms of presentation. Patients with VMD, especially patients out of childhood, have transmission defects in the lesion. Some patients appear to have subtle leaks as would be seen in chronic central serous chorioretinopathy. It is unknown whether these are actual leaks or if there is diffusion of fluorescein into the lesion with inadequate removal by incompetent RPE cells. In later stages of the disease, patients may have flat placoid areas of fibrous metaplasia of the RPE, and these areas show late staining. In some eyes the RPE metaplasia is prominent enough to suggest the presence of choroidal neovascularization.

In lesions with layering of yellowish material in the subretinal space, the superior fluid appears transparent and colorless on fundus photography and has no reflectivity during OCT. The yellow material is hyperreflective on OCT and appears as accumulations adherent to the outer retina in regions of copious subretinal fluid and sandwiched between the retina and RPE if there is not much fluid. Subretinal fluid appears to be a constant finding in VMD2, and its presence can help suggest the diagnosis [2].

The yellowish subretinal material in vitelliform lesions is intensely hyperautofluorescent. The yellowish material seen during the vitelliruptive stages is also hyperautofluorescent, but the intervening regions are not. More advanced lesions show loss of autofluorescence centrally with an increased amount of autofluorescence at the outer border of the ovoid lesion, which is usually asymmetrically distributed around the center of the macula. The material at the outer borders can have a radiating fractal or globular appearance. The centrally clearing regions show a lack of autofluorescence originating from the outer retina. The underlying RPE may have a granular autofluorescence appearance or may be devoid of autofluorescence. These regions have little or no accumulation on OCT.

There is limited histopathologic information concerning VMD. O'Gorman et al. examined the eyes of a 69-year-old donor [21]. The subretinal accumulation seen was composed of outer segment material, melanin granules, and "lipofuscin-like" material. They hypothesized that some of the retinal pigment epithelial cells degenerated and released their contents into the subretinal space. Frangieh et al. examined the eyes of an 80-year-old donor who had bilateral choroidal neovascularization and a family history of VMD [22]. The diagnosis of VMD did not appear to be confirmed in the propositus. Premorbid examination of the donor's eyes did not demonstrate any yellow subretinal material, and the gross specimens did not show any subretinal deposition of yellow material. Weingeist et al. examined the globes of a 28-year-old man with a known history of VMD, including abnormal EOG results [23]. The patient had advanced disease with concomitant areas of choroidal neovascularization. The authors noted a retinal detachment, which they thought was artifactitiously detached. Because the retina was detached, the authors only looked at the RPE and choroid with electron microscopy. Therefore, no analysis can be done of their findings of the subretinal space, which were not reported. The RPE cells contained large amounts of lipofuscin, however.

Given the lack of suitable histopathologic material, we are forced to use imaging to help determine the anatomic and physiologic conditions associated with the accumulation of subretinal material in eyes with VMD. We know that the RPE cells have increased amounts of lipofuscin in eyes with VMD. The autofluorescent material in the RPE is derived mainly from indigestible components of phagocytosed photoreceptor outer segments. Precursors of A2E, such as A2PE-H_2, A2PE, and all-*trans*-dimers, which are also autofluorescent, form in outer segments prior to phagocytosis by the RPE (Fig. 17.31) [17]. Intravitreal administration of A2PE-H_2 leads to the formation of increased amounts of A2-PE and A2E. These precursors in both central serous chorioretinopathy and VMD are thought to increase in amount through the combination of mounting accumulation of shed outer segments in the subretinal space and the prolonged duration of the accumulating material, allowing increased reaction products to form. Because of the lack of direct apposition of the photoreceptor outer segments with the RPE and the inherent delay in phagocytosis, greater yields of A2-PE by the reaction product of ATR and phosphatidylethanolamine are possible. In addition, A2E and its precursors are potentially susceptible to oxidative damage [62–65] and capable of entering into photo-oxidative reactions with neighboring molecules. Eventual phagocytosis of these older outer segments, with the degenerated material accumulating over time, would load the RPE cells with materials that are known precursors to lipofuscin and may explain why lipofuscin is found in large amounts in the RPE in VMD. A2E, oxidized metabolites of A2E, and collaterally damaged molecules are all toxic and may contribute to the high rate of visually significant complications seen in these patients, such as atrophy and choroidal neovascularization.

Somewhat similar to patients with central serous chorioretinopathy, patients with VMD have subretinal fluid. The extent of the subretinal fluid increases with the age of the patient. The source of the subretinal fluid may be related to the underlying defect in VMD2, which involves bestrophin, a Ca^{2+}-sensitive Cl^- channel protein found in the basolateral portion of the RPE cells. Mutations in the protein lead to reduced or abolished membrane current. This defect may directly or indirectly alter the ability of the RPE cells to pump fluid from the subretinal space, or it may affect the integrity of the outer blood–retinal barrier. More chronic VMD lesions have central clearing of the yellowish material, with a corresponding decrease in the observed subretinal collections seen during OCT and decreased autofluorescence from the center of the macula. In general, the accumulation of material probably reflects a dynamic process of creation and removal. In the later stages of disease, patients have obvious subretinal fluid separating the subretinal material and the RPE, making a simple increase in the rate of removal seem unlikely as the sole explanation for the decrease in yellowish material seen. In addition, these patients often have decreased visual acuity and color perception, lending credence to the possibility that the decreased amount of subretinal material in advanced cases is secondary to the decreased production of outer segments secondary to an induced atrophy. Some of these patients have patchy hyperautofluorescence from the level of the RPE, suggesting that atrophy of the underlying RPE may occur in parallel, but not strictly so.

17.15
Summary

There are many seemingly disparate diseases that cause the accumulation of autofluorescent material on the outer retina and in the subretinal space. The clinically visible manifestation of this material is yellow or yellow-orange collections. The matter may induce a color cast to the retina, with or without associated focal cream-colored dots that probably represent macrophages. In other diseases there appears to be a frank accumulation of material to produce a vitelliform deposit. The stimulus for development in many of these conditions is the physical separation of the outer retina from the RPE, making normal phagocytosis of the outer segments, a process dependent on intimate apposition, not possible [68–75].

The reason some diseases cause only a modest accumulation while other diseases are associated with a large amount of material is probably manifold. There are often lesser amounts of material in the acute phase, with accumulation over time until atrophy begins to develop. The rate of outer segment production and shedding is controlled by mechanisms that are incompletely characterized. Perturbation of the photoreceptor–RPE complex may affect the function of these cells in more than one way to contribute to the accumulation of material in the subretinal space. In addition to improper phagocytosis induced by physical separation, there may be increased outer segment production or shedding. Because there are diseases and conditions affecting RPE barrier and pump function, there may also be diseases that independently or concurrently affect the RPE's ability to phagocytose outer segments, creating the possibility of increased accumulation of outer-segment-derived material without there being a fluid-filled separation of the RPE and the overlying retina.

References

1. Spaide RF, Klancnik JM Jr. Fundus autofluorescence and central serous chorioretinopathy. Ophthalmology. 2005;112:825–833

2. Spaide RF, Noble K, Morgan A, Freund KB. Vitelliform macular dystrophy. Ophthalmology. 2006;113:1392–1400

3. Warburton S, Southwick K, Hardman RM, et al. Examining the proteins of functional retinal lipofuscin using proteomic analysis as a guide for understanding its origin. Mol Vis. 2005;11:1122–1134

4. Nilsson SE, Sundelin SP, Wihlmark U, Brunk UT. Aging of cultured retinal pigment epithelial cells: oxidative reactions, lipofuscin formation and blue light damage. Doc Ophthalmol. 2003;106:13–16

5. Kaemmerer E, Schutt F, Krohne TU, Holz FG, Kopitz J. Effects of lipid peroxidation-related protein modifications on RPE lysosomal functions and POS phagocytosis. Invest Ophthalmol Vis Sci. 2007;48:1342–1347

6. Katz ML, Drea CM, Eldred GE, et al. Influence of early photoreceptor degeneration on lipofuscin in the retinal pigment epithelium. Exp Eye Res. 1986;43:561–753

7. Katz ML, Eldred GE, Robison WG Jr. Lipofuscin autofluorescence: evidence for vitamin A involvement in the retina. Mech Ageing Dev. 1987;39:81–90

8. Eldred GE, Katz ML. Fluorophores of the human retinal pigment epithelium: separation and spectral characterization. Exp Eye Res. 1988;47:71–86

9. Bui TV, Han Y, Radu RA, et al. Characterization of native retinal fluorophores involved in biosynthesis of A2E and lipofuscin-associated retinopathies. J Biol Chem. 2006;281:18112–18119

10. Fishkin NE, Sparrow JR, Allikmets R, Nakanishi K. Isolation and characterization of a retinal pigment epithelial cell fluorophore: an all-trans-retinal dimer conjugate. Proc Natl Acad Sci USA 2005;102:7091–7096

11. Finnemann SC, Leung LW, Rodriguez-Boulan E. The lipofuscin component A2E selectively inhibits phagolysosomal degradation of photoreceptor phospholipid by the retinal pigment epithelium. Proc Natl Acad Sci USA 2002;99:3842–3847

12. Hoppe G, Marmorstein AD, Pennock EA, Hoff HF. Oxidized low density lipoprotein-induced inhibition of processing of photoreceptor outer segments by RPE. Invest Ophthalmol Vis Sci. 2001;42:2714–2720

13. Hoppe G, O'Neil J, Hoff HF, Sears J. Products of lipid peroxidation induce missorting of the principal lysosomal protease in retinal pigment epithelium. Biochim Biophys Acta. 2004;1689:33–41

14. Hoppe G, O'Neil J, Hoff HF, Sears J. Accumulation of oxidized lipid-protein complexes alters phagosome maturation in retinal pigment epithelium. Cell Mol Life Sci. 2004;61:1664–1674

15. Edwards RB, Szamier RB. Defective phagocytosis of isolated rod outer segments by RCS rat retinal pigment epithelium in culture. Science. 1977;197:1001–1003

16. Mata NL, Weng J, Travis GH. Biosynthesis of a major lipofuscin fluorophore in mice and humans with ABCR-mediated retinal and macular degeneration Proc Natl Acad Sci USA 2000;97:7154–7159

17. Liu J, Itagaki Y, Ben-Shabat S, et al. The biosynthesis of A2E, a fluorophore of aging retina, involves the formation of the precursor, A2-PE, in the photoreceptor outer segment membrane. J Biol Chem. 2000;275:29354–29360

18. Vollrath D, Feng W, Duncan JL, et al. Correction of the retinal dystrophy phenotype of the RCS rat by viral gene transfer of Mertk. Proc Natl Acad Sci USA 2001;98:12584–12589

19. Allikmets R, Singh N, Sun H, et al. A photoreceptor cell-specific ATP-binding transporter gene (ABCR) is mutated in recessive Stargardt macular dystrophy.Nat Genet. 1997;15:236–246

20. Gass JDM. Stereoscopic atlas of macular disease, 4th edn. St. Louis, Mosby, 1997, pp 60–61

21. O'Gorman S, Flaherty WA, Fishman GA, Berson EL. Histopathologic findings in Best's vitelliform macular dystrophy. Arch Ophthalmol 1988;106:1261126–12661128

22. Frangieh GT, Green WR, Fine SL. A histopathologic study of Best's macular dystrophy. Arch Ophthalmol 1982;100:1115–1121

23. Weingeist TA, Kobrin JL, Watzke RC. Histopathology of Best's macular dystrophy. Arch Ophthalmol 1982;100:1108–1114

24. Arnold JJ, Sarks JP, Killingsworth MC, Kettle EK, Sarks SH. Adult vitelliform macular degeneration: a clinicopathological study. Eye. 2003;17:717–26

25. Dubovy SR, Hairston RJ, Schatz H, et al. Adult-onset foveomacular pigment epithelial dystrophy: clinicopathologic correlation of three cases. Retina. 2000;20:638–649

26. Eckardt C, Eckardt U, Groos S, et al. Macular translocation in a patient with adult-onset foveomacular vitelliform dystrophy with light- and electron-microscopic observations on the surgically removed subfoveal tissue. Graefes Arch Clin Exp Ophthalmol. 2004;242:456–467

27. Shields JA, Rodrigues MM, Sarin LK, et al. Lipofuscin pigment over benign and malignant choroidal tumors. Trans Sect Ophthalmol Am Acad Ophthalmol Otolaryngol. 1976;81:871–881

28. Takagi T, Tsuda N, Watanabe F, Noguchi S. Subretinal precipitates of retinal detachments associated with intraocular tumors. Ophthalmologica. 1988;197:120–126

29. Spaide RF, Campeas L, Haas A, et al. Central serous chorioretinopathy in younger and older adults. Ophthalmology 1996;103: 2070–2080

30. Wang M, Sander B, Lund-Andersen H, Larsen M. Detection of shallow detachments in central serous chorioretinopathy. Acta Ophthalmol Scand. 1999;77:402–405

31. Eandi CM, Chung JE, Cardillo-Piccolino F, Spaide RF. Optical coherence tomography in unilateral resolved central serous chorioretinopathy. Retina 2005;25:417–421

32. Anderson DH, Stern WH, Fisher SK, Erickson PA, Borgula GA. Retinal detachment in the cat: the pigment epithelial-photoreceptor interface. Invest Ophthalmol Vis Sci. 1983;24:906–926

33. Kaplan MW, Iwata RT, Sterrett CB. Retinal detachment prevents normal assembly of disk membranes in vitro. Invest Ophthalmol Vis Sci. 1990;31:1–8

34. Hale IL, Fisher SK, Matsumoto B. Effects of retinal detachment on rod disc membrane assembly in cultured frog retinas. Invest Ophthalmol Vis Sci. 1991;32:2873–2881

35. Williams DS, Fisher SK. Prevention of rod disk shedding by detachment from the retinal pigment epithelium. Invest Ophthalmol Vis Sci. 1987;28:184–187

36. Matsuo T. Photoreceptor outer segments in aqueous humor: key to understanding a new syndrome. Surv Ophthalmol. 1994;39:211–233

37. Iida T, Spaide RF, Haas A, et al. Leopard-spot pattern of yellowish subretinal deposits in central serous chorioretinopathy. Arch Ophthalmol 2002;120:37–42

38. Spaide RF. Deposition of yellow submacular material in central serous chorioretinopathy resembling adult-onset foveomacular vitelliform dystrophy. Retina. 2004;24:301–304

39. Eandi CM, Sugin S, Spaide RF. Descending atrophic tracts associated with choroidal hemangioma. Retina. 2005;25:216–218

40. Brown GC, Shields JA, Goldberg RE. Congenital pits of the optic nerve head. II. Clinical studies in humans. Ophthalmology 1980;87:51–65

41. Sugar, HS. Congenital pits in the optic disc with acquired macular pathology. Am J Ophthalmology 1962; 53:307–311

42. Gass JDM. Serous detachment of the macular secondary to congenital pit of the optic nerve head. Am J Ophthalmol 1969;67: 821–841

43. Ie D, Yannuzzi LA, Spaide RF, Rabb MF, Blair NP, Daily MJ. Subretinal exudative deposits in central serous chorioretinopathy. Br J Ophthalmol. 1993;77:349–353

44. Gass JD. Idiopathic senile macular hole. Its early stages and pathogenesis. Arch Ophthalmol. 1988;106:629–639

45. Machemer R. Experimental retinal detachment in the owl monkey. IV. The reattached retina. Am J Ophthalmol 1968;66:1075–1091

46. Robertson DM. Delayed absorption of subretinal fluid after scleral buckling procedures: the significance of subretinal precipitates. Trans Am Ophthalmol Soc. 1978;76:557–583

47. Kaga T, Fonseca RA, Dantas MA, Yannuzzi LA, Spaide RF. Optical coherence tomography of bleb-like subretinal lesions after retinal reattachment surgery. Am J Ophthalmol. 2001;132:120–121

48. Hagimura N, Iida T, Suto K, Kishi S. Persistent foveal retinal detachment after successful rhegmatogenous retinal detachment surgery. Am J Ophthalmol. 2002;133:516–520

49. Panozzo G, Parolini B, Mercanti A. OCT in the monitoring of visual recovery after uneventful retinal detachment surgery. Semin Ophthalmol. 2003;18:82–84

50. Gass JD, Chuang EL, Granek H. Acute exudative polymorphous vitelliform maculopathy. Trans Am Ophthalmol Soc. 1988;86:354–366

51. Chan CK, Gass JD, Lin SG. Acute exudative polymorphous vitelliform maculopathy syndrome. Retina. 2003;23:453–462

52. Cruz-Villegas V, Villate N, Knighton RW, Rubsamen P, Davis JL. Optical coherence tomographic findings in acute exudative polymorphous vitelliform maculopathy. Am J Ophthalmol. 2003;136:760–763

53. Sotodeh M, Paridaens D, Keunen J, et al. Paraneoplastic vitelliform retinopathy associated with cutaneous or uveal melanoma and metastases. Klin Monatsbl Augenheilkd. 2005;222:910–914

54. Marmorstein AD, Marmorstein LY, Rayborn M, et al. Bestrophin, the product of the Best vitelliform macular dystrophy gene (VMD2), localizes to the basolateral plasma membrane of the retinal pigment epithelium. Proc Natl Acad Sci USA 2000;97:12758–12763

55. Sun H, Tsunenari T, Yau KW, Nathans J. The vitelliform macular dystrophy protein defines a new family of chloride channels. Proc Natl Acad Sci USA 2002;99:4008–4013

56. Seddon JM, Afshari MA, Sharma S, et al. Assessment of mutations in the Best macular dystrophy (VMD2) gene in patients with adult-onset foveomacular vitelliform dystrophy, age-related maculopathy, and bull's-eye maculopathy. Ophthalmology 2001;108:2060–2067

57. Jarc-Vidmar M, Kraut A, Hawlina M. Fundus autofluorescence imaging in Best's vitelliform dystrophy. Klin Monatsbl Augenheilkd 2003;220:861–867

58. Gass JDM. Stereoscopic atlas of macular diseases. Diagnosis and treatment. Mosby, St. Louis; 1997, pp 304–311

59. Deutman AF, Hoyng CB. Macular Dystrophies. In Ryan SJ, ed. Retina, 3rd edn. Mosby, St. Louis; 2001, pp 1210–1257

60. Chung JE, Spaide RF. Fundus autofluorescence and vitelliform macular dystrophy. Arch Ophthalmol 2004;122:1078–1079

61. Spaide RF, Klancnik Jr JM. Fundus autofluorescence and central serous chorioretinopathy. Ophthalmology 2005;112:825–833

62. Dillon J, Wang Z, Avalle LB, Gaillard ER. The photochemical oxidation of A2E results in the formation of a 5,8,5',8'-bis-furanoid oxide. Exp Eye Res 2004;79:537–542

63. Sparrow JR, Zhou J, Ben-Shabat S, et al. Involvement of oxidative mechanisms in blue-light-induced damage to A2E-laden RPE. Invest Ophthalmol Vis Sci 2002;43:1222–1227

64. Kim SR, Nakanishi K, Itagaki Y, Sparrow JR. Photooxidation of A2-PE, a photoreceptor outer segment fluorophore, and protection by lutein and zeaxanthin. Exp Eye Res. 2006;82:828–839

65. Sparrow JR, Boulton M. RPE lipofuscin and its role in retinal pathobiology. Exp Eye Res. 2005;80:595–606

66. Katz ML, Robison WG Jr. Age-related changes in the retinal pigment epithelium of pigmented rats. Exp Eye Res. 1984;38:137–151

67. Edwards RB. Stimulation of rod outer segment phagocytosis by serum occurs only at the RPE apical surface. Exp Eye Res. 1991;53:229–232

68. Ryeom SW, Sparrow JR, Silverstein RL. CD36 participates in the phagocytosis of rod outer segments by retinal pigment epithelium. J Cell Sci. 1996;109(Pt 2):387–395

69. Nguyen-Legros J, Hicks D. Renewal of photoreceptor outer segments and their phagocytosis by the retinal pigment epithelium. Int Rev Cytol. 2000;196:245–313

70. Finnemann SC. Focal adhesion kinase signaling promotes phagocytosis of integrin-bound photoreceptors. EMBO J. 2003;22:4143–4154

71. Nandrot EF, Finnemann SC. Altered rhythm of photoreceptor outer segment phagocytosis in beta5 integrin knockout mice. Adv Exp Med Biol. 2006;572:119–123

72. Hall MO, Obin MS, Heeb MJ, et al. Both protein S and Gas6 stimulate outer segment phagocytosis by cultured rat retinal pigment epithelial cells. Exp Eye Res. 2005;81:581–591

73. Nandrot EF, Anand M, Sircar M, Finnemann SC. Novel role for alphaVbeta5-integrin in retinal adhesion and its diurnal peak. Am J Physiol Cell Physiol. 2006;290:C1256–C1262

74. Sun M, Finnemann SC, Febbraio M, et al. Light-induced oxidation of photoreceptor outer segment phospholipids generates ligands for CD36-mediated phagocytosis by retinal pigment epithelium: a potential mechanism for modulating outer segment phagocytosis under oxidant stress conditions. J Biol Chem. 2006;281:4222–4230

75. Akeo K, Hiramitsu T, Yorifuji H, Okisaka S. Membranes of retinal pigment epithelial cells in vitro are damaged in the phagocytotic process of the photoreceptor outer segment discs peroxidized by ferrous ions. Pigment Cell Res. 2002;15:341–347

76. Spaide RF, Fisher Y, Ober M, Stoller G. Surgical hypothesis: Inner retinal fenestration as a treatment for optic disc pit maculopathy. Retina. 2006;26:89–91

Fig. 17.1 Autofluorescence originating from the outer retina and subretinal space links a number of seemingly disparate diseases

Increased Autofluorescence from the Retina and Subretinal Space

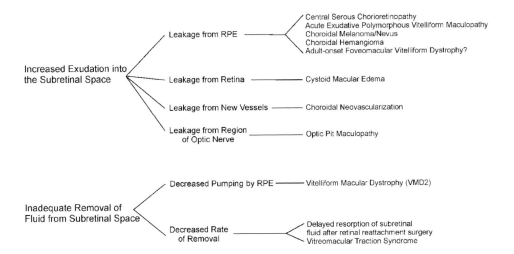

Increased Exudation into the Subretinal Space

Leakage from RPE
- Central Serous Chorioretinopathy
- Acute Exudative Polymorphous Vitelliform Maculopathy
- Choroidal Melanoma/Nevus
- Choroidal Hemangioma
- Adult-onset Foveomacular Vitelliform Dystrophy?

Leakage from Retina — Cystoid Macular Edema

Leakage from New Vessels — Choroidal Neovascularization

Leakage from Region of Optic Nerve — Optic Pit Maculopathy

Inadequate Removal of Fluid from Subretinal Space

Decreased Pumping by RPE — Vitelliform Macular Dystrophy (VMD2)

Decreased Rate of Removal
- Delayed resorption of subretinal fluid after retinal reattachment surgery
- Vitreomacular Traction Syndrome

Fig. 17.2 **a** This patient had an acute leak, and when imaged 2 months after the beginning of his symptoms (**b**), showed minimal changes in autofluorescence. When imaged 3 months later, the gravitating material in the subretinal space blocked the background choroidal fluorescence (**c**), and the area of detachment was hyperautofluorescent (**d**). One month after the photographs **c** and **d** were taken, the patient had another autofluorescent photograph (**e**), which showed an increase in the autofluorescence. Note the accumulation of material on the outer retina as seen by optical coherence tomography (**f**). Eight months after presentation, which was 1 month following spontaneous resolution of the patient's symptoms, the retina was flat, and much of the diffuse hyperautofluorescence had resolved, leaving aggregates of hyperautofluorescence (**g**). Optical coherence tomography (**h**) taken through the central portion of the previously detached retina in the same location and orientation as the scan shown in image **d** shows that much of the subretinal accumulation has been resorbed, leaving focal mounds of material (*arrows*) (From Spaide RF, Klancnik JM Jr. Fundus autofluorescence and central serous chorioretinopathy. Ophthalmology. 2005;112:825–833)

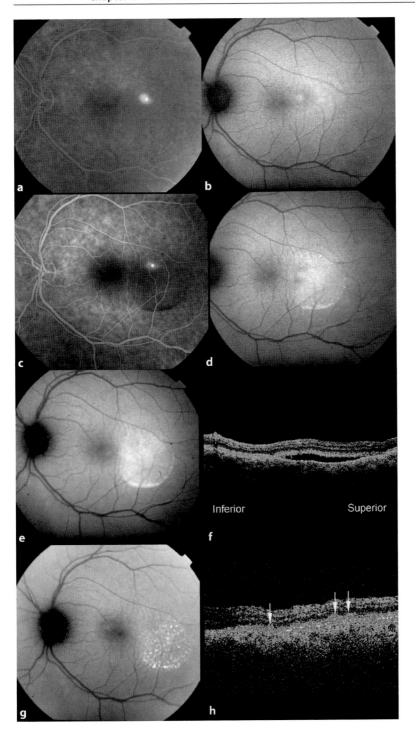

Fig. 17.3a,b A comparison of the autofluorescence photograph of the serous detachment with the autofluorescence photograph shows that the dots of hyperautofluorescence correspond to punctate subretinal precipitates as seen in the color photograph. These punctate dots are seen in central serous chorioretinopathy and a number of other diseases and are thought to be lipofuscin-laden macrophages on the outer surface of the retina. (From Spaide RF, Klancnik JM Jr. Fundus autofluorescence and central serous chorioretinopathy. Ophthalmology. 2005;112:825–833)

Fig. 17.4 The left eye had subretinal fluid from central serous chorioretinopathy, but the fluid has resolved. There are subretinal flecks of yellow material (*arrows*) and an area of noncentral geographic atrophy (*arrowhead*) (**a**). In the autofluorescence photograph, the yellow flecks appear hyperautofluorescent and the noncentral geographic atrophy appears hypoautofluorescent. The visual acuity was 20/30

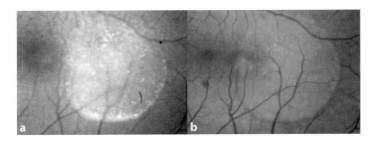

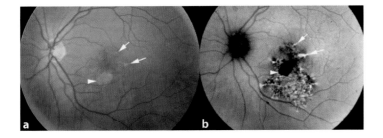

Fig. 17.5 a,b Comparison of the right and left eyes shows that the area of detachment caused by central serous chorioretinopathy is frankly yellow. **c,d** Green monochromatic photographs highlight the differences in reflectivity between the two eyes. **e,f** The serous detachment is hyperautofluorescent. **g** Optical coherence tomography shows a thick accumulation of material on the outer surface of the retina

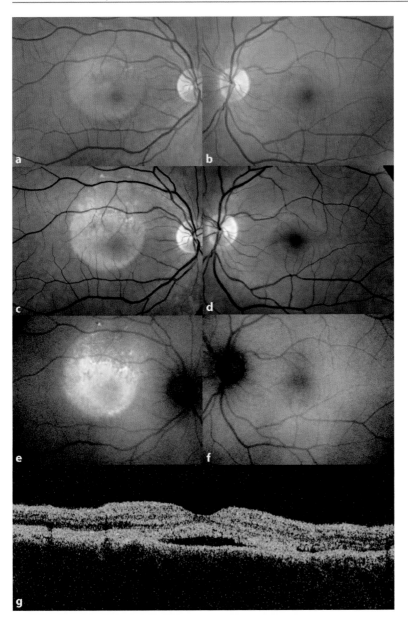

Fig. 17.6 a This patient was being treated with corticosteroids and developed chronic central serous chorioretinopathy. Note the large accumulation of yellowish subretinal material, which was evident on green monochromatic photography (**b**). The fluorescein angiogram (**c**) shows chronic leakage with blocking by the overlying yellow material

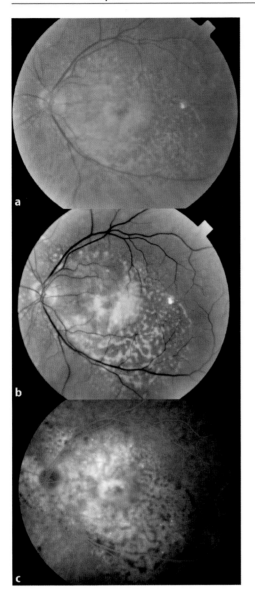

17.7 This patient had chronic subretinal fluid in the macular region and relative hypoautofluorescence centrally. The accumulation on the outer retina was relatively thin. The visual acuity was 20/40

Fig. 17.8 This patient had chronic central serous chorioretinopathy leading to severely decreased acuity in the right eye. In his left eye he had chronic subretinal fluid in the nasal macula but recently had increasing symptoms associated with an increase in the amount of subretinal fluid. Note the recent advent of the descending tracts, which are largely hyperautofluorescent. (From Spaide RF, Klancnik JM Jr. Fundus autofluorescence and central serous chorioretinopathy. Ophthalmology. 2005;112:825–833)

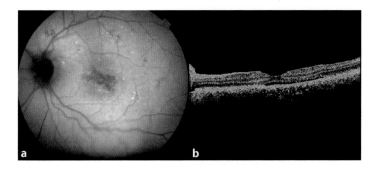

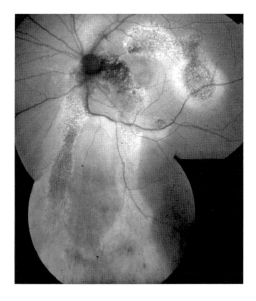

Fig. 17.9 Proposed mechanism of subretinal autofluorescence in central serous chorioretinopathy. **a** The leak causes a circumscribed elevation of the macula. **b** The elevated retina is no longer in contact with the retinal pigment epithelium. Shed photoreceptors are not phagocytosed. **c** Increasing accumulation of degenerated, shed photoreceptors creates an increasing amount of reaction products that are autofluorescent. Macrophages invade the area, attempting to phagocytose the accumulated material. **d** With chronic detachment the photoreceptors eventually atrophy, leading to a decrease in the subretinal accumulation. Note the concurrent atrophy of the underlying retinal pigment epithelium

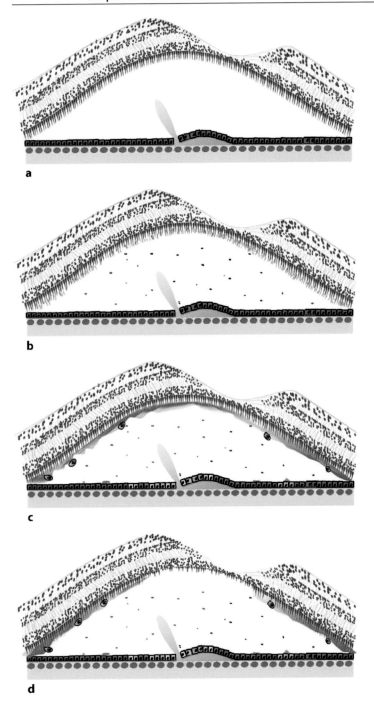

Fig. 17.10 This 68-year-old man had a 6-month history of central serous chorioretinopathy before this examination. **a** He had a serous neurosensory detachment of the macula (*arrows*) and a small amount of yellow submacular material (*arrowhead*). **b** He had a leak at the level of the retinal pigment epithelium in the temporal macula. **c** There was persistence of the leak when the patient was examined 1.5 years later, with increased accumulation of yellow submacular material (**d**). When examined 5.5 years after presentation, the patient continued to have a large unilateral ovoid area of submacular material similar to that seen in adult-onset foveomacular vitelliform dystrophy (**e**) (Modified from Spaide RF. Deposition of yellow submacular material in central serous chorioretinopathy resembling adult-onset foveomacular vitelliform dystrophy. Retina. 2004;24:301–304)

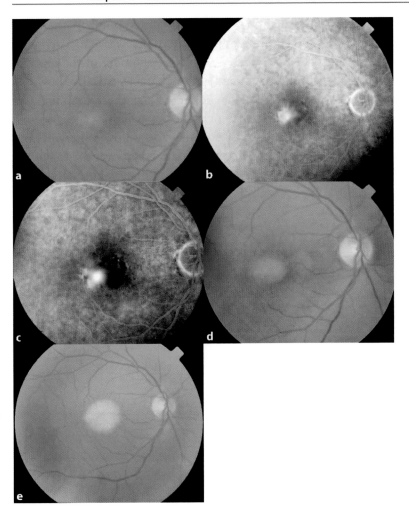

Fig. 17.11 a A choroidal hemangioma located superotemporal to the optic nerve head has the typical reddish-orange appearance. This was associated with yellowish subretinal material (*arrow*) and a serous detachment of the macula. **b** The earliest frames of the fluorescein angiogram characteristically show filling of vascular channels within the hemangioma. **c** Later there is staining of the hemangioma, and the yellow pigment blocks the hyperfluorescence (*arrow*). **d** Autofluorescence photography demonstrates that the yellow material is hyperautofluorescent. **e** An optical coherence tomogram taken over the top of the tumefaction shows the subretinal fluid and granules of material in the subretinal space (*arrow*)

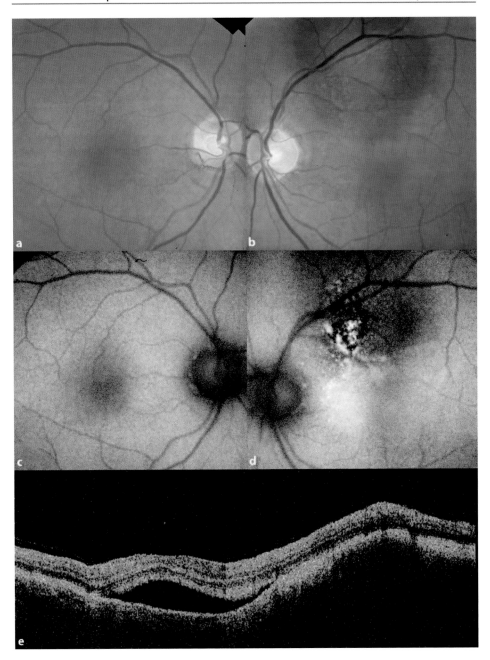

Fig. 17.12 a,b Right and left eyes of a patient with a melanocytic lesion in the left eye. Note the dependent serous detachment of the macula in the left eye that has a slight yellow cast. There is orange subretinal material over the tumefaction. **c,d** The autofluorescence photographs of the right and left eyes show increased autofluorescence in the area of the detachment and focal hyperautofluorescent spots, corresponding to orange material. **e** A composite optical coherence tomogram shows the dependent serous detachment with accumulation of subretinal material in the region of the detachment

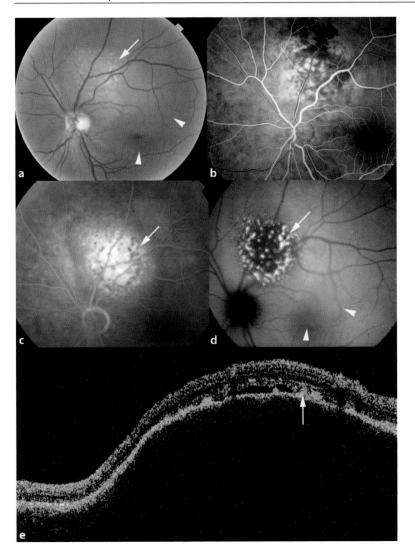

Fig. 17.13 a,b This patient had pseudophakic cystoid macular edema in the left eye, causing a slight increase in autofluorescence from the central fovea. **c** Note the accumulation of subretinal material under the central fovea

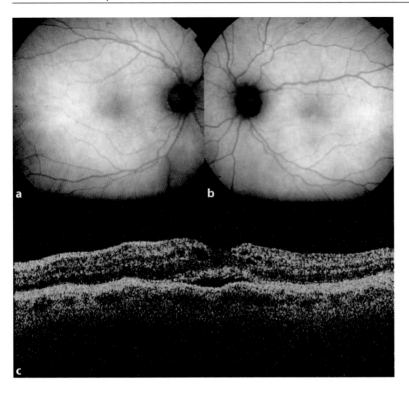

Fig. 17.14 **a** The color photograph shows an area of choroidal neovascularization under the macula and a nevus superotemporal to the macula. The patient had yellow deposits commonly lumped together under the term "lipid." Note the differing appearance of the lipid. **b** Autofluorescence photography shows decreased autofluorescence over the nevus with focal areas of hyperautofluorescence. The macular lesion has decreased autofluorescence centrally, as seen in cases of long-standing choroidal neovascularization. Note the differential autofluorescence appearance of the two types of "lipid"

Fig. 17.15 Close-up of Fig. 17.13. The *arrows* point to a fine granular intraretinal accumulation similar to that seen in diabetic retinopathy. Inferiorly there are spheroidal blobs of yellowish outer retinal accumulation. **b** The autofluorescence photograph shows hypoautofluorescence from the intraretinal lipid (*arrows*). The outer retinal accumulations are hyperautofluorescent. The *arrows* point to lipoproteins associated with increased leakage of serum components, while the spheroidal accumulations may represent material derived from shed photoreceptor outer segments

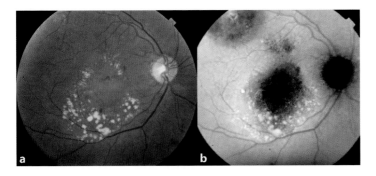

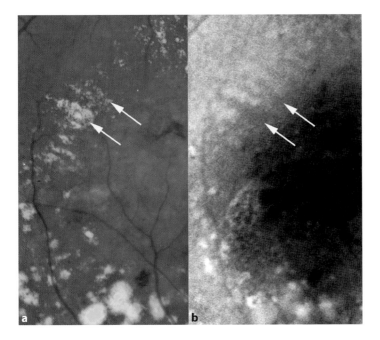

Fig. 17.16 a,b A 7-year-old girl was referred for evaluation of the serous macular detachment of the left eye. She had experienced dimness of vision of the affected eye for 1 year. Visual acuity was 20/20 in the right eye and 20/30 uncorrected in the left eye. An optic pit was located at the inferotemporal border of the optic disk of the left eye, with a shallow neurosensory macular detachment tapering toward the optic pit with yellowish subretinal precipitates. **c** A higher magnification view demonstrates the slight yellow cast of the area of detachment with focal accumulations of yellow material. **d** Autofluorescence photography demonstrates increased autofluorescence in the area of detachment with hyperautofluorescent subretinal accumulations. **e** Optical coherence tomography shows an outer-layer retinal detachment noncontiguous to the optic disc. There were hyperreflective accumulations of material on the outer part of the retina (*arrow*). **e** Optical coherence tomography shows an outer-layer retinal detachment noncontiguous to the optic disc. There were hyperreflective accumulations of material on the outer part of the retina (*arrow*). (From Laud K, Visaetsilpanonta S, Yannuzzi LA, Spaide RF. Autofluorescence imaging of optic pit maculopathy. Retina. 2007;27:116–119)

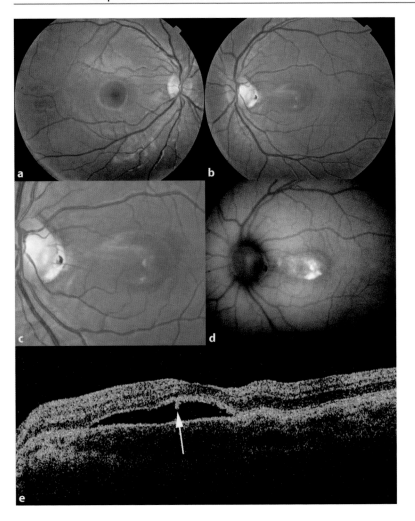

Fig. 17.17 a,b The right eye of a 26-year-old architect had an optic nerve pit at the border of an optic disc much larger than the fellow eye. The optic nerve pit was associated with a macular detachment containing yellow material. The visual acuity was 20/60. **c,d** The yellow material was hyperautofluorescent. **e** The outer surface of the detachment had a shaggy accumulation of material (From K, Visaetsilpanonta S, Yannuzzi LA, Spaide RF. Autofluorescence imaging of optic pit maculopathy. Retina. 2007;27:116–119)

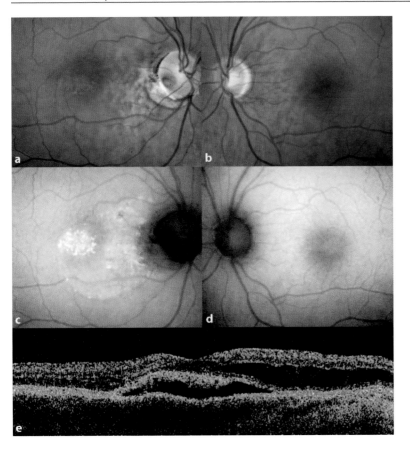

Fig. 17.18 The patient in Fig. 17.16 underwent an outer retinal fenestration [76]. **a** When examined 2 months later the detachment had resolved, although there was still some inner retinal edema. Note the decrease in yellow material with a corresponding decrease in the associated hyperautofluorescence (**b**). **c** The optical coherence tomogram shows cystoid changes in the inner retina, but a flattening of the detachment

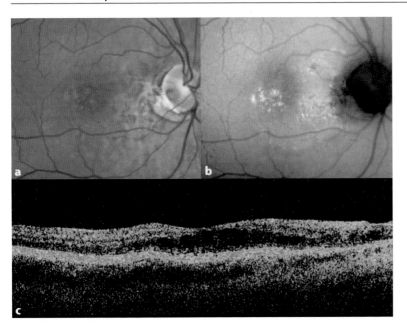

Fig. 17.19 a This patient had vitreomacular traction syndrome. **b** An optical coherence tomographic picture taken after vitrectomy shows a collection of subretinal fluid with material on the outer surface of the retina. **c** One year later the patient had a yellow spot in the center of the macula in the right eye. **d** The left eye had no similar abnormality. **e** Autofluorescence photography shows a hyperautofluorescent area corresponding to the accumulation seen in image **c**. **f** The optical coherence tomographic picture shows a mound of material under the central fovea. The patient was examined 1 year later, and there was no change in the yellow hyperautofluorescent spot in the right eye. Note that if the patient had been examined without a history, the appearance of the right macula might have suggested the diagnosis of adult-onset foveomacular vitelliform dystrophy

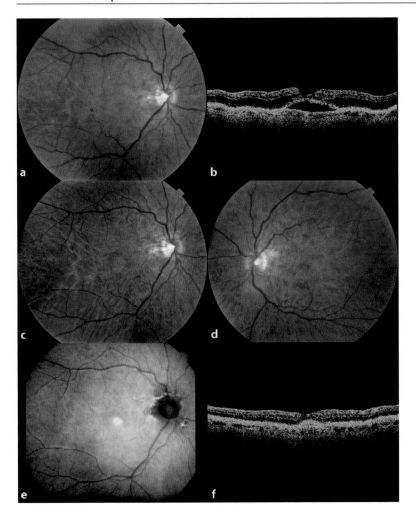

Fig. 17.20a–c This patient had a small yellow dot in the center of the fovea consistent with a stage 1 macular hole of Gass. The autofluorescence photograph shows a hyperautofluorescent spot. The optical coherence tomographic picture photograph shows increased accumulation on the outer surface of the foveola (**c**). In this case, the stage 1 macular hole appearance actually corresponded to what Gass proposed before the existence of optical coherence tomography, which is not true for many patients with prehole states. The origin of the observed yellow color may be from the accumulated material on the outer surface of the retina

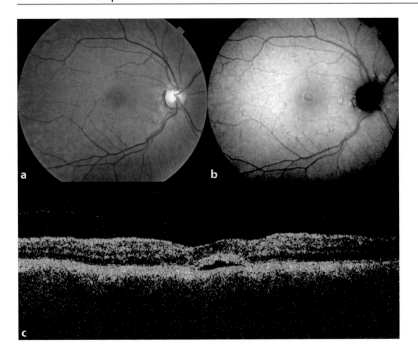

Fig. 17.21 a This patient had prominent vitreomacular traction with a small amount of hemorrhage above the central macular detachment. **b** Optical coherence tomography shows a dramatic picture of traction and elevation of the central macula. **c** The patient underwent vitrectomy and membrane peeling. The detachment partially flattened, leaving a collection of yellow material superior to the fovea when examined 1 week after surgery. Note that the yellow dots on the outer surface of the retina appear much the same as those seen in central serous chorioretinopathy. **d** The optical coherence tomographic scan shows persistent subretinal fluid and a hyperreflective thickening at the outer retina corresponding to the yellow material. **e** The autofluorescence photograph taken on the same day shows that both the yellow material and the punctate dots are hyperautofluorescent. **f** One month later there was partial reabsorption of the yellow material superiorly. **g** Four months later there was partial resolution of the subretinal fluid. The yellow dots are in a different position than in image **c**, and the dots were hyperautofluorescent

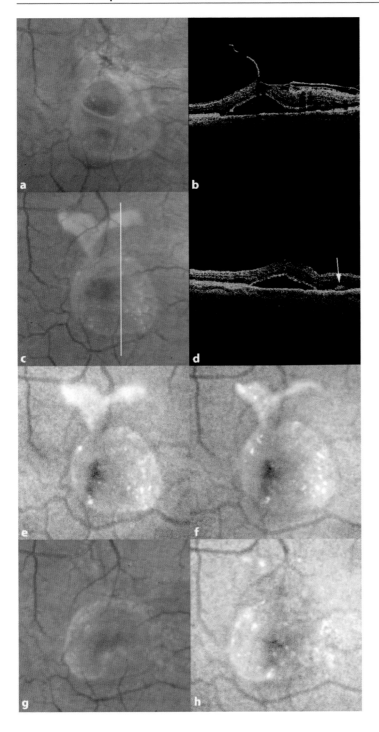

Fig. 17.22 **a** This 67-year-old had a retinal detachment repaired with cryopexy and a 360° buckle. He had flattening of the retina with persistence of subretinal fluid under the fovea of the right eye. The monochromatic photograph shows the fovea in the right eye to be lighter that the fovea in the left. **c,d** The right eye showed slight hyperautofluorescence of the central macula in the right eye as compared with the left. **e** Optical coherence tomography shows accumulation of material on the outer retina in the area of detachment

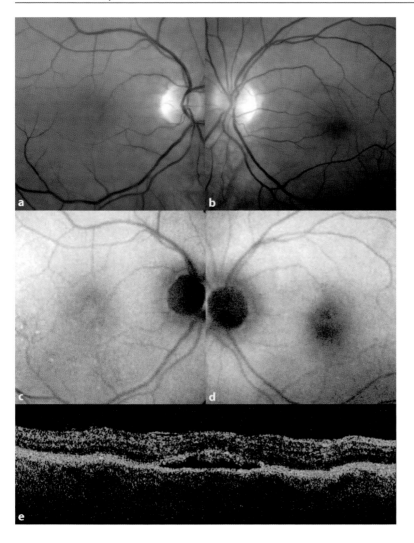

Fig. 17.23 **a,b** Six months after the photograph in Fig. 17.22 was taken, the patient had a more discrete light spot in the center of the fovea in the right eye as compared with the left. **c,d** The yellow material was hyperautofluorescent. **e** Optical coherence tomography showed that the yellow material corresponded to an accumulation in the subretinal space. If the right eye had been examined without knowledge of the previous ocular history, a diagnosis of adult-onset foveomacular dystrophy would have been considered

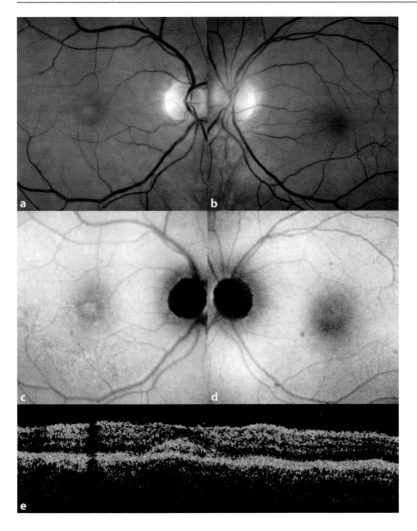

Fig. 17.24 **a,b** This patient had an acute loss of visual acuity secondary to acute exudative polymorphous vitelliform maculopathy. The color photograph demonstrates the bilateral subretinal collections of yellowish material formed with resorption of the subretinal fluid. There are numerous discrete blebs superiorly. The central macula had a collapse of the subretinal material to form a gravitating accumulation of a large amount of the yellow material inferiorly, while the superior macula is relatively devoid of the material. **c,d** The overall background choroidal fluorescence was decreased, but the yellowish material blocked the background choroidal fluorescence. **e,f** The yellowish material was highly autofluorescent

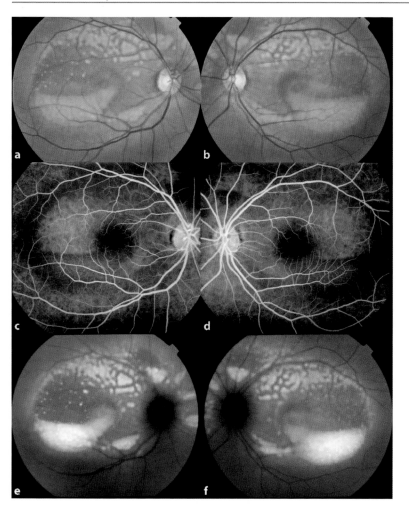

Fig. 17.25 **a** This 47-year-old-woman, the mother of the patient in Fig. 17.26, had an abnormal electro-oculogram that was measured after her daughter was diagnosed with vitelliform macular dystrophy type 2. Based on the family history, the mother was an obligate carrier. She did not have any abnormalities as noted by red-free photography (**a**), fluorescein angiography (**b**), autofluorescence photography (**c**), or optical coherence tomography (**d**)

Fig. 17.26 **a** This 14-year-old patient had a typical vitelliform lesion. **b** The deposition of the yellowish material was not homogeneous within the lesion, as seen by red-free monochromatic photography. **c** The autofluorescence photograph shows hyperautofluorescence of the material with the same pattern seen in image **b**. **d** Optical coherence tomography shows deposition of material on the outer retina with a clear subretinal space below. (From Spaide RF, Noble K, Morgan A, Freund KB. Vitelliform macular dystrophy. Ophthalmology. 2006;113:1392–1400)

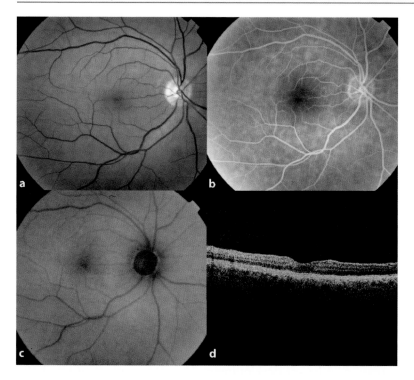

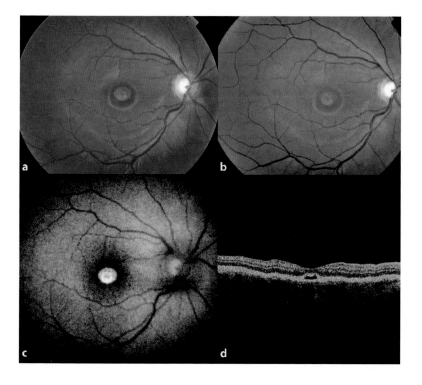

Fig. 17.27 a,b This 6.5-year-old with vitelliform macular dystrophy type 2 had deposition of yellowish material in the macular region of both eyes. Note that the material is not uniformly distributed and that there are areas where the material is denser. **c,d** The autofluorescence photographs taken on a prototype system show increased autofluorescence corresponding to the denser areas of deposition seen in the red-free monochromatic pictures. (From Spaide RF, Noble K, Morgan A, Freund KB. Vitelliform macular dystrophy. Ophthalmology. 2006;113:1392–1400)

Fig. 17.28 Progression of lesion development. The same patient in Fig. 17.27 is shown 4 years later. **a** The macular lesion is larger. The color photograph alludes to the complexity of the lesion. There is a fluid level (*large arrow*) with yellowish material in the inferior portion of the lesion and relatively transparent fluid superiorly. In the superior portion of the lesion, alteration in the color at the level of the retinal pigment epithelium (RPE) is evident (*small arrow*). The visual acuity was 20/25. **b** The red-free monochromatic photograph shows the fluid level between the yellowish material and the relatively transparent fluid superiorly. It does not resolve the whitish placoid change at the level of the RPE seen in image **a**. **c** Fluorescein angiography shows increased fluorescence superiorly in the lesion and blocking inferiorly by the yellowish material. There was very slight leakage of fluorescein in the course of the fluorescein examination. **d** The autofluorescence photograph shows that the yellow material was intensely autofluorescent but that the placoid change at the level of the RPE was not. The photographic findings of images **a–d** suggest that the placoid change was fibrous metaplasia of the RPE, although neovascularization may be present as well. **e** An optical coherence tomography (OCT) scan taken vertically shows the dependent deposition of material in the subretinal space (*arrows*). **f** An OCT scan taken horizontally through the fovea shows a shaggy accumulation of material on the outer retina with underlying fluid that has no reflectivity (From Spaide RF, Noble K, Morgan A, Freund KB. Vitelliform macular dystrophy. Ophthalmology. 2006;113:1392–1400)

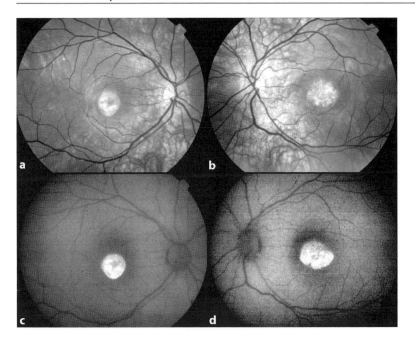

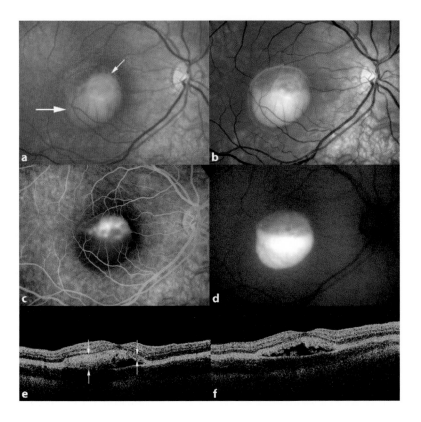

Fig. 17.29 The father of the patient shown in Figs. 17.27 and 17.28. **a** The right eye had an almost complete absence of the yellowish subretinal material except at the outer edges of the lesion. In the central portion of the lesion, there was what appeared to be fibrous metaplasia of the retinal pigment epithelium (RPE). The visual acuity was 20/50. **b** The fluorescein angiogram shows staining centrally with slight leakage of fluorescein into the inferior portions of the lesion. **c** The autofluorescence photograph shows a relative lack of autofluorescence centrally, with hyperautofluorescence in the periphery of the lesion corresponding to the material seen in image **a**. **d** Optical coherence tomography shows elevation of the macula by subretinal fluid. There is an accumulation of material on the outer retina (*arrows*). The material has almost no thickness in the central macula and becomes thicker at the edges of the retinal elevation. There is an elevation at the level of the RPE (*arrowhead*), which may represent RPE metaplasia (From Spaide RF, Noble K, Morgan A, Freund KB. Vitelliform macular dystrophy. Ophthalmology 2006;113:1392–1400)

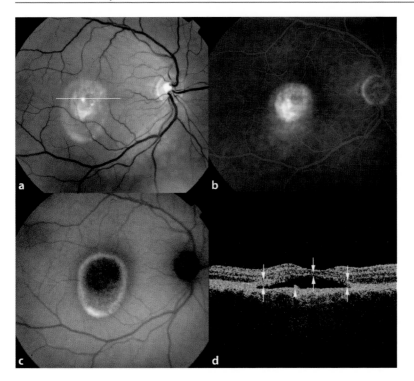

Fig. 17.30 a Color photography of a 42-year-old with vitelliform macular dystrophy type 2 shows the asymmetrical distribution of the lesion around the macula with the dependent extension of the lesion inferiorly. The visual acuity was 20/80. **b** The yellowish material at the outer border is hyperautofluorescent, and there is a lack of autofluorescence centrally. **c,d** The early- and late-phase fluorescein angiographic pictures show the transmission defects within the lesion and the suggestion of late staining and subtle leakage present. **e** Optical coherence tomography done horizontally through the superior macula (as shown in image **a**) illustrates the macular elevation by subretinal fluid. Note that the material on the outer retina is thin centrally and thicker at the edges of the lesion (*arrows*) (From Spaide RF, Noble K, Morgan A, Freund KB. Vitelliform macular dystrophy. Ophthalmology. 2006;113:1392–1400)

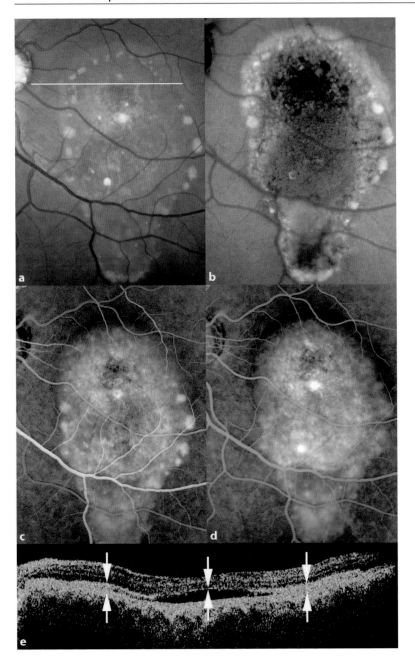

Fig. 17.31 Proposed pathophysiologic changes in vitelliform macular dystrophy type 2 (VMD2). Eyes with VMD2 uniformly have subretinal fluid as seen by optical coherence tomography. The physical separation of the retina from the retinal pigment epithelium (RPE) would prevent proper apposition of the outer segments with the RPE. Shed but nonphagocytosed outer segments could build up in the subretinal space. Infiltrating this material could be macrophages. There is no intrinsic mechanism to prevent the formation of A2-PE-H$_2$, A2-PE, all-*trans*-dimers, and other precursors to A2E in the degenerating outer segments. The shed outer segments could eventually make their way to the RPE, but the phagocytosed material would theoretically load the RPE cells with the precursors to A2E and also oxidized lipids and proteins. The toxic effect of this material may cause RPE atrophy, metaplasia, and choroidal neovascularization

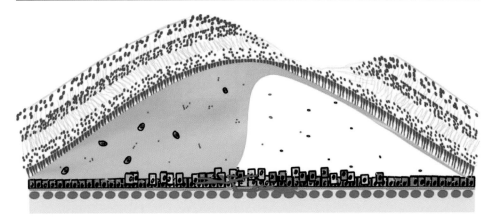

18.1
Macular Holes

Full-thickness macular holes are associated with corresponding markedly increased intensity in autofluorescence (Fig. 18.1) [5, 7, 15, 23]. In the absence of neurosensory retina, there is also no luteal pigment. Hence, the excitation and emission light can directly pass to and from the uncovered retinal pigment epithelium (RPE). The affected area also corresponds well to hyperfluorescence seen with fluorescein angiography. By optical coherence tomography, the edges of the macular hole are often upturned, presenting an increased thickness for the excitation light to pass through, which may explain the decreased autofluorescence intensity sometimes seen surrounding the hole. The attached operculum in stage 2 macular holes and the preretinal operculum in stage 3 macular holes show a focally decreased autofluorescence from blocking.

Following successful surgical treatment, the area with increased autofluorescence disappears, and almost normal or normal distribution of autofluorescence is seen. Partial-thickness macular holes are usually associated with an increased fundus autofluorescence (FAF) signal, whereby the degree increment depends on the amount of luteal pigment left in the remaining neurosensory retinal tissue.

18.2
Foveal Hypoplasia

Isolated foveal hypoplasia is considered a rare congenital condition [6, 18]. Fundus changes such as an absent or abnormal maculofoveal reflex and distinct capillary alterations in the central macula may be only very subtle, and it may be difficult to diagnose this cause of poor central visual function. Optical coherence tomography is helpful in establishing the diagnosis [13, 14]. Because of the absence of macular luteal pigment, FAF imaging in patients with foveal hypoplasia shows no decreased intensity, but rather normal background signal in the central area (Fig. 18.2).

18.3
Chloroquine Maculopathy

Kellner and colleagues demonstrated that FAF imaging may show distinct alterations in patients taking chloroquine/hydroxychloroquine medication [9]. A pericentral ring of increased intensity was present in patients with mild changes. More advanced stages showed a more mottled appearance with levels of increased and decreased intensity in the pericentral macula (Fig. 18.3). Electrophysiology is thought to remain the most sensitive tool to diagnose early chloroquine maculopathy. However, FAF imaging appears to be more sensitive than fundus photograph or fluorescein angiography in detecting toxic alterations at the level of the RPE.

18.4
Optic Disc Drusen

Optic disc drusen have autofluorescent properties and can be readily visualized by a bright nodular autofluorescence (Fig. 18.4) [10, 16, 17]. Drusen buried within the nerve may be more visible by autofluorescence photography than by ophthalmoscopy, although deeply buried disc drusen may require B-mode ultrasonography for detection. Optic nerve drusen are highly associated with nerve fiber layer loss and visual field defects [8, 21]. It is unknown whether the drusen or the nerve fiber layer defect is the primary defect.

18.5
Pseudoxanthoma Elasticum

Pseudoxanthoma elasticum (PXE) has a prevalence of 1 in 25,000 and causes abnormalities chiefly involving the eye, skin, and cardiovascular system [4]. The gene defect in PXE has been characterized as a loss of function mutation in the ATP-binding cassette subtype C number 6 gene (ABCC6) [2, 11, 20]. The function of the protein encoded by this gene is not known, but it is probably a transport protein. ABCC6 is in the same superfamily as the ABCA4 mutation which causes Stargardt disease [1, 22].

PXE can cause angioid streaks, which appear as hypoautofluorescent fissures; optic nerve drusen, which are intensely autofluorescent; and peau d' orange, which causes a subtle granular stippling (Fig. 18.5). More serious complications include RPE atrophy, the extent of which was not appreciated prior to autofluorescence imaging, as well as choroidal neovascularization (CNV). Patients with PXE can have RPE atrophy that generally falls into three categories: large cracks that look like rips, multilobular areas of discrete atrophy, and diffuse poorly defined regions of atrophy (Fig. 18.5). In some patients the atrophy is preceded by hyperautofluorescent flecks or spots. CNV can be recognized by its typical features during autofluorescence photography. The potential ingrowth of CNV may be potentiated in PXE by the angioid streaks and the RPE atrophy [22].

18.6
Bilateral Diffuse Uveal Melanocytic Proliferation

Patients with bilateral diffuse uveal melanocytic proliferation have proliferation of benign melanocytes in the outer choroid; this proliferation is histopathologically un-related to the primary non-ocular carcinoma [24]. These patients also develop nu-merous round or oval areas of loss of RPE cells. Fluorescein angiography shows these nummular areas to be transmission defects, autofluorescence photography shows them to be devoid of autofluorescence, and optical coherence tomography reveals them to have no visible cellular elements at the level of the RPE (Fig. 18.6). This loss of RPE cells has been attributed to a paraneoplastic process.

18.7
Congenital Hypertrophy of the Retinal Pigment Epithelium

Congenital hypertrophy of the RPE (CHRPE) is a hyperpigmented, generally flat le-sion with well-demarcated borders that may mimic other pigmented lesions in the eye such as ocular nevi and melanomas. The cells show hypertrophy, but they do not appear to be involved in outer segment turnover. The overlying photoreceptor cells are degenerated [3] and melanosomes are distributed uniformly in the RPE cell, but there is no lipofuscin [12, 19], and there is an absolute scotoma within the lesion. Unlike choroidal nevi, which generally have minimal autofluorescence changes un-less there is subretinal fluid or orange pigment, CHRPE lesions are markedly hypo-autofluorescent (Fig. 18.7). By comparison, choroidal melanomas frequently have hyperautofluorescent collections from orange pigment or from chronic detachment. Although the differentiation of these lesions is usually straightforward, autofluores-cence photography can supply supplemental information.

References

1. Allikmets, R, Singh, N, Sun, H, et al. (1997) A photoreceptor cell-specific ATP-binding transporter gene (ABCR) is mutated in recessive Stargardt macular dystrophy. Nat Genet 15:236–246

2. Bergen, AA, Plomp, AS, Schuurman, EJ, et al. (2000) Mutations in ABCC6 cause pseudoxanthoma elasticum. Nat Genet 25:228–231

3. Buettner, H (1975) Congenital hypertrophy of the retinal pigment epithelium. Am J Ophthalmol 79:177–189

4. Chassaing, N, Martin, L, Calvas, P, et al. (2005) Pseudoxanthoma elasticum: a clinical, pathophysiological and genetic update including 11 novel ABCC6 mutations. J Med Genet 42:881–892

5. Ciardella, AP, Lee, GC, Langton, K, et al. (2004) Autofluorescence as a novel approach to diagnosing macular holes. Am J Ophthalmol 137:956–959

6. Curran, RE, Robb, RM (1976) Isolated foveal hypoplasia. Arch Ophthalmol 94:48–50

7. Framme, C, Roider, J (2001) Fundus autofluorescence in macular hole surgery. Ophthalmic Surg Lasers 32:383–390

8. Katz, BJ, Pomeranz, HD (2006) Visual field defects and retinal nerve fiber layer defects in eyes with buried optic nerve drusen. Am J Ophthalmol 141:248–253

9. Kellner, U, Renner, AB, Tillack, H (2006) Fundus autofluorescence and mfERG for early detection of retinal alterations in patients using chloroquine/hydroxychloroquine. Invest Ophthalmol Vis Sci 47:3531–3538

10. Kurz-Levin, MM, Landau, K (1999) A comparison of imaging techniques for diagnosing drusen of the optic nerve head. Arch Ophthalmol 117:1045–1049

11. Le Saux, O, Urban, Z, Tschuch, C, et al. (2000) Mutations in a gene encoding an ABC transporter cause pseudoxanthoma elasticum. Nat Genet 25:223–227

12. Lloyd, WC, 3rd, Eagle, RC, Jr., Shields, JA, et al. (1990) Congenital hypertrophy of the retinal pigment epithelium. Electron microscopic and morphometric observations. Ophthalmology 97:1052–1060

13. McGuire, DE, Weinreb, RN, Goldbaum, MH (2003) Foveal hypoplasia demonstrated in vivo with optical coherence tomography. Am J Ophthalmol 135:112–114

14. Meyer, CH, Lapolice, DJ, Freedman, SF (2003) Foveal hypoplasia demonstrated in vivo with optical coherence tomography. Am J Ophthalmol 136:397; author reply 397–398

15. Milani, P, Seidenari, P, Carmassi, L, Bottoni, F (2007) Spontaneous resolution of a full thickness idiopathic macular hole: fundus autofluorescence and OCT imaging. Graefes Arch Clin Exp Ophthalmol

16. Mustonen, E, Nieminen, H (1982) Optic disc drusen—a photographic study. I. Autofluorescence pictures and fluorescein angiography. Acta Ophthalmol (Copenh) 60:849–858

17. Neetens, A, Burvenich, H (1977) Autofluorescence of optic disc-drusen. Bull Soc Belge Ophtalmol 179:103–110

18. Oliver, MD, Dotan, SA, Chemke, J, Abraham, FA (1987) Isolated foveal hypoplasia. Br J Ophthalmol 71:926–930

19. Parsons, MA, Rennie, IG, Rundle, PA, et al. (2005) Congenital hypertrophy of retinal pigment epithelium: a clinico-pathological case report. Br J Ophthalmol 89:920–921

20. Ringpfeil, F, Lebwohl, MG, Christiano, AM, Uitto, J (2000) Pseudoxanthoma elasticum: mutations in the MRP6 gene encoding a transmembrane ATP-binding cassette (ABC) transporter. Proc Natl Acad Sci USA 97:6001–6006

21. Roh, S, Noecker, RJ, Schuman, JS, et al. (1998) Effect of optic nerve head drusen on nerve fiber layer thickness. Ophthalmology 105:878–885

22. Sawa, M, Ober, MD, Freund, KB, Spaide, RF (2006) Fundus autofluorescence in patients with pseudoxanthoma elasticum. Ophthalmology 113:814–820 e812

23. von Rückmann, A, Fitzke, FW, Gregor, ZJ (1998) Fundus autofluorescence in patients with macular holes imaged with a laser scanning ophthalmoscope. Br J Ophthalmol 82:346–351

24. Wu, S, Slakter, JS, Shields, JA, Spaide, RF (2005) Cancer-associated nummular loss of the pigment epithelium. Am J Ophthalmol 139:933–935

Fig. 18.1 *Top row:* Red-free reflectance and fundus autofluorescence (FAF) images of the right eye of a patient with macular hole. FAF imaging shows distinct changes with a bright signal inside the hole and a surrounding ring of decreased intensity. *Bottom row:* Optical coherence tomography and schematic drawing. The edges of the hole are usually upturned, like a drawbridge. Hence, the excitation light has a larger distance to travel through the neurosensory retina to reach the retinal pigment epithelium and backward again (*arrows*). This may cause more absorption by luteal pigment and could explain the decreased autofluorescence at the edge of the hole

Fig. 18.2 Fundus photograph, optical coherence tomography (OCT), and fundus autofluorescence (FAF) images of a 24-year-old man. He had poor vision from a young age, without progressive deterioration. At presentation, visual acuities were 6/18 in both eyes. Electrophysiology showed misrouting at the chiasm, suggesting ocular albinism, while no features of cutaneous albinism were visible. Horizontal OCT scanning discloses continuous retinal layers through the central retina. In addition to the absence of the foveal avascular zone, FAF imaging shows normal background levels and no decreased intensity (lack of macula pigment) in the center of the macula. *Images courtesy of Declan Flanagan, consultant ophthalmic surgeon, Moorfields Eye Hospital, London*

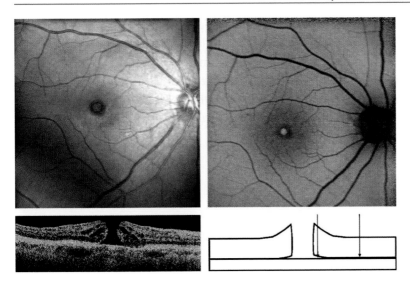

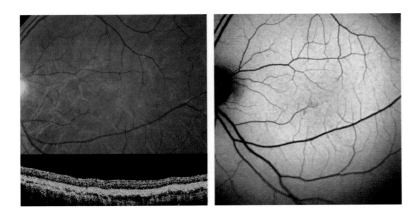

Fig. 18.3 Reflectance, optical coherence tomography (OCT), fundus autofluorescence (FAF), and late-phase fluorescein angiography images of a 51-year-old woman with chloroquine maculopathy. FAF imaging shows a mottled pattern of increased and decreased intensities in the pericentral retina and further levels of increased intensity toward eccentricity. In the fovea itself, a cystoid macula edema is present in both eyes, showing irregular levels of increased autofluorescence

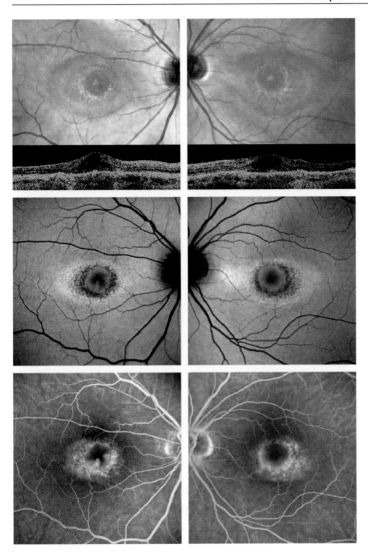

Fig. 18.4 *Top row:* Bilateral disc drusen characterized by markedly increased fundus autofluorescence (FAF) signals in the central portion of the optic disc. Large retinal arterial and venous vessels anterior to the drusen mask the FAF signal. *Middle and bottom rows:* Unilateral disc drusen in the left eye. The nerve fiber analysis demonstrates marked reduction in nerve fiber layer thickness of the left eye compared with the uninvolved right eye

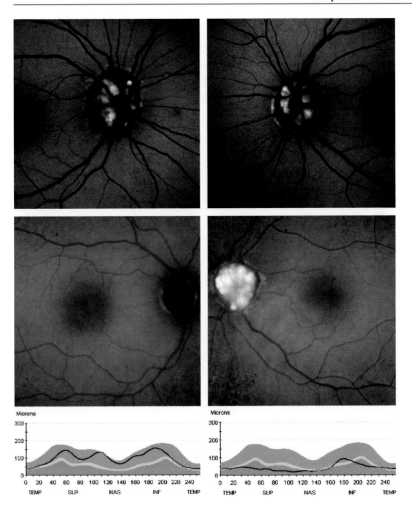

Fig. 18.5 Pseudoxanthoma elasticum. **a** A montage autofluorescence photograph shows extensive atrophy of the macula and radiating angioid streaks (*arrow*) with associated lobular areas of retinal pigment epithelium (RPE) atrophy (*arrowhead*) that resemble pearls on a string. Drusen of the optic nerve are hyperautofluorescent (*small arrow*). **b** A montage autofluorescence photograph shows extensive scarring in the macula from choroidal neovascularization, with lobular areas of atrophy (*small arrowhead*) and diffuse areas of poorly defined RPE atrophy (*large arrowhead*)

Fig. 18.6 a This patient with uterine cancer had a rapid profound loss of vision in both eyes secondary to bilateral diffuse uveal melanocytic proliferation. She had a myriad of round areas of what had been called retinal pigment epithelial atrophy in the past. **b** Fluorescein angiography showed multiple transmission defects, and the autofluorescence photograph showed a loss of the normal fundus autofluorescence in these regions of transmission defect. Optical coherence tomography revealed that the nummular areas had no cellular elements at the level of the retinal pigment epithelium (From Wu S, Slakter JS, Shields JA, Spaide RF (2005) Cancer-associated nummular loss of the pigment epithelium. Am J Ophthalmol 139:933–935)

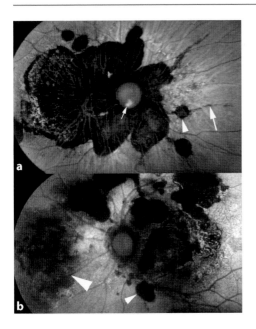

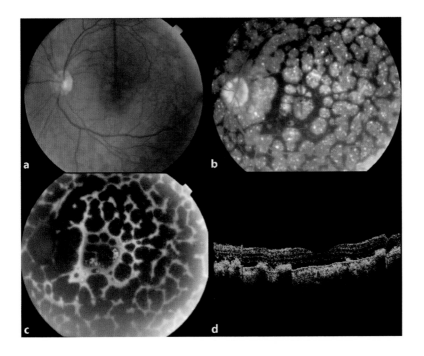

Fig. 18.7 **a** This lesion of congenital hypertrophy of the retinal pigment epithelium measures approximately 11 mm in diameter. **b** The corresponding autofluorescence photograph shows a lack of autofluorescence within the lesion, consistent with the known lack of lipofuscin within the retinal pigment epithelial cells in the lesion

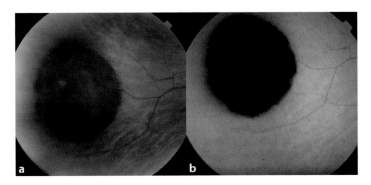

Part III
Perspectives in
Imaging Technologies

19.1
Introduction

Today, over 10 years after the first visualization of the topographic distribution of lipofuscin accumulation over larger retinal areas in vivo using confocal scanning laser ophthalmoscopy (cSLO), fundus autofluorescence imaging (FAF) is increasingly been used in research and in the clinical setting [17]. FAF findings now also serve to identify high-risk features and rapid progressors in an ongoing large interventional trial of patients with geographic atrophy secondary to age-related macular degeneration (http://www.siriontherapeutics.com).

However, there are limitations to currently used FAF imaging devices. These include resolution and quantification issues as well as distinction of different underlying fluorophores according to spectral characteristics. Novel emerging imaging techniques offer new perspectives. They may add to our current knowledge of various retinal diseases and contribute to the development of new therapeutic strategies.

19.2
Image Acquisition and Processing

Inconsistencies in findings from different research groups may to some degree originate from different imaging systems and/or different image acquisition and processing protocols. As the advantages and the clinical value of FAF imaging are better appreciated and FAF imaging is applied within multicenter trials, it is important to establish standardized operating procedures (SOP) for image acquisition and processing in order to compare and reliably analyze obtained results. The awareness of potential pitfalls during image acquisition and subsequent reading of FAF imaging (see Chap. 4) can greatly help to improve image quality and minimize inaccurate interpretation of FAF findings. For example, there is no data or consensus yet on how many single images of a cSLO series are optimal for generating the final FAF mean image. As outlined previously (see Chap. 4), this is largely dependent on the imaging protocol and processing as well as on the selected patient population. For example, the SOP of the FAM (*Fundus Autofluorescence in Age-Related Macular Degeneration*) study requires obtaining a series of at least 15 images and selecting nine single images for calculation of the mean image [14]. This represents a relatively small number of single images, but it is a practical protocol that has been reliably used in a multicenter trial.

With recent developments in image processing, including improved algorithms to more accurately align single images of a series for the correction of eye movements during acquisition, better image quality with increased single-to-noise ratio may be achieved. This may also allow use of a larger number of images. A greater number of well-aligned images for the calculation of mean images will improve the signal-to-noise ratio and therefore improve image quality. Here, the possibility to obtain mean images during the acquisition—in other words, in real time—has already been realized in a commercially available system (Heidelberg Retina Angiography and Spectralis OCT) and is a major step forward, but further investigation is needed.

Following the calculation of the mean image, the pixel values within the FAF image are usually normalized in order to better visualize the distribution of autofluorescence intensities for the human eye (see Chap. 4). This image-processing step usually helps to evaluate FAF findings. However, the current algorithm in available systems may cause difficulties in the interpretation of levels of decreased FAF in certain pathological conditions. Non-normalized mean images can be used to manually adjust the pixel distribution of a certain area with decreased intensities, such as in the fovea. Therefore, it is already possible today to visualize different structures within these areas for the eye of the grader. However, a more standardized approach or a more sophisticated algorithm is required to overcome obscuring of details within areas of a markedly decreased signal.

19.3
Quantification of the FAF Signal

The FAF image shows the spatial distribution of the intensity of the FAF signal for each pixel in gray values. By definition, pixel grey values are categorized on an arbitrary scale from 0 to 255. These values can be used for numeric calculations and subsequent statistical analyses of FAF intensities. Using pixel grey values, several authors have consistently reported that FAF imaging permits reliable evaluation of the relative distribution of the FAF signal over the posterior pole. Typical ratios between the intensity of the fovea and the perifoveal macula have been established in normal subjects (see Chaps. 6 and 7). Based on these findings, qualitative descriptions of localized FAF changes are widely used. Usually, the FAF signal over a certain retinal location is categorized in decreased, normal, or increased intensities in comparison to the background signal of the same image.

In contrast, the quantification of absolute intensities and their comparison between subjects or within longitudinal observation in the same subject is by far more complicated and remains a challenge in the context of FAF imaging. It must be emphasized that pixel values of processed and normalized images are not absolute and therefore must not be used for such analyses. Of note, the image processing software in commercially available systems easily allows the operator to turn off this modification and to calculate the mean image without the normalization of pixel values. Furthermore, it should be noted that the digital resolution of the detector in current imaging devices exceeds the maximum spatial resolution of ocular media and the optics of the system (see Chap. 4). Therefore, single pixel values of a standard FAF image do not reflect the actual anatomical resolution of the image. They should not be used to compare intensities between different locations. When pixel values are used for topographic FAF intensity calculation, the actual image resolution has to be taken into account, and it would be more appropriate to summarize the values of a certain group of neighboring pixels rather than to use single pixel values.

For analysis of absolute intensities on non-normalized FAF images, there is already a great variability of the mean grey value for a certain retinal location when two observers subsequently acquire the FAF image from the same subject directly one after the other using the same imaging device. The interobserver reproducibility was only moderate in one study comparing the absolute mean pixel value of a 16×16-pixel square on the retina, which would encompass a reasonable large retinal area of about 2×1.9° [7]. Several considerations must be taken into account when comparing absolute FAF intensities between different examinations and different patients. First, settings such as laser power, detector sensitivity, correction of refractive errors, and image processing steps (including the number of averaged images) must be standardized. Second, eye movements, the position of the patient in the chin rest, the axial orientation of the camera, and the distance between the camera and the cornea can all potentially influence the illumination of the fundus and can cause subtle differences in the magnitude of pixel values within the FAF image. Third, the laser power or the flash of the excitation light varies slightly over time. The manufacturer recommends not acquiring images before turning on the laser for a certain period. This will usually ensure achieving a reasonable stability of the laser power for standard FAF imaging. Fourth, individual variances between subjects, such as refractive error and optic media (above all, lens status), will have an impact on the FAF intensity. Particularly, nuclear yellowing and advanced cataract can greatly absorb the excitation light (see Chap. 4.7). This will cause artificial low intensities and may affect the distribution of the signal over the whole fundus. Fifth, the FAF signal and distribution might be slightly altered by dynamic metabolic processes of the accumulation of lipofuscin in the retinal pigment epithelium (RPE). Circadian rhythms, dark adaption of the patient's eye, or bleaching effects by previous prolonged exposure to the blue excitation light may represent confounding factors for the absolute quantification of the FAF signal.

Although some of these factors may be standardized at least for longitudinal observations of the same subject, most of them will still influence quantitative FAF intensities to a considerable extent. Before pixel values are used for absolute calculation and comparison of FAF intensities between images, refinement of the imaging technology of current available systems appears to be mandatory. Until a high reproducibility of obtained pixel values and their distribution is ensured, pixel values should not be used for quantitative analysis of FAF intensities.

19.4

Color Imaging of the Fundus Using the cSLO

The cSLO represent the most widely used imaging device for FAF imaging, and most FAF findings have been obtained with the cSLO. Compared with the traditional fundus camera system, main advantages of the cSLO include the confocal setup with the ability to detect FAF signals from the layer of interest and largely overcome lens fluorescence, the imaging of large retinal areas, and high sensitivity with enhanced image contrast. Furthermore, FAF images with the cSLO can be obtained without exposing the retina to the high levels of illumination required for FAF imaging with the fundus camera. Despite these advances, one of the limitations of commercially available cSLO systems for FAF imaging is the inability to obtain a fundus color image. Color images represent the imaging gold standard for documenting various fundus changes (e.g., drusen appearance) and are helpful, even sometimes mandatory, for interpretation of FAF findings.

Because the cSLO uses a laser as excitation light, it primarily records monochromatic images. By combining low-power red, green, and blue laser reflectance images, realistic color SLO images can be produced—analogous to the formation of color television images using red, green, and blue phosphors [1, 3, 8, 11]. Imaging devices with rapid pulsing of the laser and hence illumination of each retinal point by three colors in quick succession have produced the acquisition of quasisimultaneous color SLO fundus images. It should be noted that these images reflect the fundus reflectance of a discrete spectrum instead of the continuous spectrum of the white flash light of the fundus camera. Due to the different imaging principle, comparison with conventional color fundus photographs is limited, and it has not been systematically evaluated yet.

Obtaining FAF images and true color SLO imaging with one-imaging devices has not been reported yet. Such an SLO system may not only be beneficial and more practical for documenting fundus changes but may also help quantify FAF intensities.

19.5

Metabolic Mapping of Additional Fluorophores

Lipofuscin represents the dominant fluorophores of the ocular fundus, detected by FAF imaging with the established excitation and emission wavelengths. In addition to lipofuscin, the visualization of minor fluorophores at the ocular fundus might be of interest in studying ocular disease or even—considering the eye as the window of the body—in identifying and monitoring systemic disorders as well [10, 15, 16, 18]. Minor fluorophores include NAD- NADH$^+$ (oxidized and reduced nicotinamidadenindinucleotide) and FAD-FADH² (oxidized and reduced flavinadeninucleotide). These re-dox pairs act as electron carriers in oxidative phosphorylation in mitochondria and would potentially allow determination of the partial pressure of oxygen in ocular tissue. Advanced glycation end-products, collagen, and elastin also have autofluorescent properties, and the visualization of their topographic distribution may serve as a diagnostic tool or identify prognostic determinants in degenerative diseases.

Several limitations have to be overcome to image the autofluorescence intensity in these potential candidates, including the very weak fluorescence signal, the separation from the relatively stronger signal of lipofuscin, and the influence of the crystalline lens.

19.6
Adaptive Optics

As mentioned earlier (Chap. 3), the lateral resolution with current available imaging systems is limited by the numerical aperture and high-order aberrations of the ocular media. The latter can be corrected by the use of adaptive optics [4, 9, 12, 13]. This technique was originally introduced to overcome blur in ground-based telescopes and has recently been used to image individual cellular structures, including the photoreceptor mosaic in the mammalian eye in vivo. Combining confocal detection, autofluorescence imaging, multispectral imaging, and adaptive optics, Gray and colleagues were able to image the polygonal pattern of RPE cells in the living monkey macula [4]. The visualization of fine-detail structures with adaptive optics, including RPE morphology, is a very promising step forward in retinal imaging. Its application in large patient populations and its implementation in nonexperimental imaging systems are still warranted.

19.7
Two-Photon Excited Fluorescence Imaging

Confocal fluorescence microscopy has been a revolution in imaging of fine structures within thick tissue. By utilizing pinholes to exclude out-of-focus background fluorescence from detection, the effective sensitivity of the layer of interest is greatly increased. With the use of a scanning laser system in which a laser beam scans the image in x and y directions, a digital high-resolution image can be constructed. The application of this technology in ophthalmology led to the development of the cSLO and the ability to visualize lipofuscin accumulation at the RPE in the living eye and its changes in certain retinal diseases. However, certain limitations must be taken into account when obtaining fluorescence images with confocal optics. Because the pinholes block most of the emitted light, the exciting light must be very bright to allow an adequate signal-to-noise ratio. As subsequent scans are made, the bright light can cause fluorescent dyes to fade, or toxic free radicals can be generated by the excited fluorescence. When imaging the human ocular fundus, it is important to take not only maximal permissible exposure levels into account but also the influence of the ocular media. In addition to the limited penetration depth by absorption of light throughout the beam path, both the excitation and the emission photons are scattered by the tissue in the light beam. Scattered light originating from nonretinal structures is not entirely blocked by the pinhole of the confocal system and can therefore reach the detector, adding to the background noise.

In two-photon excited fluorescence imaging, fluorescence is not generated by a single photon as in conventional techniques, but by two lower-energy photons that both interact with the fluorophore and are absorbed in a very short interval. Focusing the laser beam of a femtosecond laser that exhibits very short, intense pulses of about 10^{-5} s, a significant number of two-photon absorption events at the point of interest is achieved. The combination of effectively concentrating the excitation energy spatially and in time ensures that the average laser power remains fairly low and that no large amounts of background noise are generated from the beginning. Further advantages of two-photon excited fluorescence include the use of infrared instead of blue excitation light. The longer wavelength of infrared light results in less energy, less phototoxicity, and less scattered light. Overall, compared with current single-photon SLO systems, two-photon excited fluorescence may therefore potentially result in better signal-to-noise ratio and better image contrast, permitting the visualization of more and deeper retinal structures.

The imaging possibilities of two-photon excited fluorescence in ophthalmology were recently demonstrated on human postmortem ocular tissue [2]. The morphology of RPE cells and the individual distribution of lipofuscin granules were clearly visualized and age-dependent differences investigated (Fig. 19.1). Taking advantage

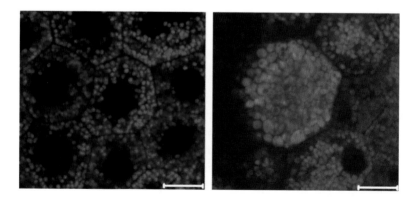

Fig. 19.1 Illustration of changes in retinal pigment epithelium cell morphology and lipofuscin distribution with age in human donor eyes in the macula area using two-photon excited fluorescence microscopy after Bindewald-Wittich et al. [2]. The *left* image shows a regular hexagonal pattern in 19-year-old donor eyes with small lipofuscin granules at the cellular borders. In contrast, the pattern is disorganized, and increased accumulation of lipofuscin granules can be observed in a 55-year-old donor eye (*right*). In the latter, single cells with densely packed, large lipofuscin granules are visualized thanks to the large sensing depth of two-photon excited fluorescence

of other retinal fluorophores (see above), photoreceptor outer segments with the cone and rod mosaic, tissue fibers within Bruch's membrane, and extracellular deposits and blood cells in the choriocapillaris were studied without slicing or cutting through the neurosensory retina.

The implementation of two-photon excited fluorescence in the scanning laser ophthalmoscope system for application in vivo may also permit visualization of the topographic lipofuscin distribution with improved signal-to-noise ratio, larger sensing depth, and greater detail. Here, safety issues of the femtosecond laser coupled to the scanning laser system must be addressed and retinal damage threshold values defined before application in the human eye [5, 6].

References

1. Ashman, RA, Reinholz, F, Eikelboom, RH (2001) Improvements in colour fundus imaging using scanning laser ophthalmoscopy. Lasers Med Sci 16:52–59

2. Bindewald-Wittich, A, Han, M, Schmitz-Valckenberg, S, et al. (2006) Two-photon-excited fluorescence imaging of human RPE cells with a femtosecond Ti:sapphire laser. Invest Ophthalmol Vis Sci 47:4553–4557

3. Fitzke, FW (1998) Colour imaging using a scanning laser ophthalmoscope. Br J Ophthalmol 82:337–338

4. Gray, DC, Merigan, W, Wolfing, JI, et al. (2006) In vivo fluorescence imaging of primate retinal ganglion cells and retinal pigment epithelial cells. Opt Express 14:7144–7158

5. Konig, K, Ehlers, A, Riemann, I, et al. (2007) Clinical two-photon microendoscopy. Microsc Res Tech

6. König, K, So, PTC, Mantulin, WW, Gratton, E (1997) Cellular response to near-infrared femtosecond laser pulses in two-photon microscopes. Optics Letters 22:135–136

7. Lois, N, Halfyard, AS, Bunce, C, et al. (1999) Reproducibility of fundus autofluorescence measurements obtained using a confocal scanning laser ophthalmoscope. Br J Ophthalmol 83:276–279

8. Manivannan, A, Van der Hoek, J, Vieira, P, et al. (2001) Clinical investigation of a true color scanning laser ophthalmoscope. Arch Ophthalmol 119:819–824

9. Miller, DT, Williams, DR, Morris, GM, Liang, J (1996) Images of cone photoreceptors in the living human eye. Vision Res 36:1067–1079

10. Nelson, DA, Krupsky, S, Pollack, A, et al. (2005) Special report: noninvasive multi-parameter functional optical imaging of the eye. Ophthalmic Surg Lasers Imaging 36:57–66

11. Reinholz, F, Ashman, RA, Eikelboom, RH (1999) Simultaneous three wavelength imaging with a scanning laser ophthalmoscope. Cytometry 37:165–170

12. Romero-Borja, F, Venkateswaran, K, Roorda, A, Hebert, T (2005) Optical slicing of human retinal tissue in vivo with the adaptive optics scanning laser ophthalmoscope. Appl Opt 44:4032–4040

13. Roorda, A, Williams, DR (1999) The arrangement of the three cone classes in the living human eye. Nature 397:520–522

14. Schmitz-Valckenberg, S, Jorzik, J, Unnebrink, K, Holz, FG (2002) Analysis of digital scanning laser ophthalmoscopy fundus autofluorescence images of geographic atrophy in advanced age-related macular degeneration. Graefes Arch Clin Exp Ophthalmol 240:73–78

15. Schweitzer, D, Hammer, M, Schweitzer, F, et al. (2004) In vivo measurement of time-resolved autofluorescence at the human fundus. J Biomed Opt 9:1214–1222

16. Schweitzer, D, Schenke, S, Hammer, M, et al. (2007) Towards metabolic mapping of the human retina. Microsc Res Tech

17. von Ruckmann, A, Fitzke, FW, Bird, AC (1995) Distribution of fundus autofluorescence with a scanning laser ophthalmoscope. Br J Ophthalmol 79:407–412

18. Winkler, BS, Pourcho, RG, Starnes, C, et al. (2003) Metabolic mapping in mammalian retina: a biochemical and 3H-2-deoxyglucose autoradiographic study. Exp Eye Res 77:327–337

Subject Index

A

A2E   242
- biosynthesis   5
- drusen   22
- functional correlate   149
- light   9
- photooxidation   7
- RPE cell damage   9
- spectrum   4, 21
- structure   4
ABCA4   5, 10, 243, 314
abnormal phenotype   80, 98
acute exudative polymorphous vitelliform maculopathy   251
acute posterior multifocal placoid pigment epitheliopathy   208
acute syphilitic posterior placoid chorioretinitis   209
acute zonal occult outer retinopathy   212
adaptive optics   19, 33, 335
adult-onset vitelliform dystrophy   9, 88, 90, 247, 252. *see also* Best disease
Age-Related Eye Disease Study (AREDS)   65
artefact   43

B

Best disease   9, 86, 252
Bietti crystalline corneoretinal dystrophy   114
birdshot chorioretinopathy   213
bleaching effect   333

C

cartwheel pattern   166
cataract   47
causes for an increased FAF signal   73
causes for a reduced FAF signal   72
central serous chorioretinopathy   245
chloroquine maculopathy   314
choroidal tumor   248
chromatic aberration   38, 41
classification   149
- early AMD   135
- FAF phenotyping   135
- GA secondary to AMD   149
cone-rod dystrophy   104, 121
cone dystrophy   104, 106
confocal optic   31, 335
convex hull   158
cSLO
- acquisition process   38
- excitation energy   31
- filter   33
- light level   37
- systems   33
- technical details   33

D

dark choroid   79
diabetic maculopathy   75
dominant drusen   92
doyne honeycomb maculopathy   92
drusen   22
- confluent   134
- crystalline   134